PREGN
THE NA
WAY

Dr Sarah Brewer MA, MB, BChir

SOUVENIR PRESS

First published 1999 by
Souvenir Press Ltd,
43 Great Russell Street, London WC1B 3PA

ISBN 0 285 63511 5

Typeset by Rowland Phototypesetting Ltd,
Bury St Edmunds, Suffolk

Printed in Great Britain by
The Guernsey Press Company Ltd,
Guernsey, Channel Islands

Contents

CONTENTS

Foreword

A woman experiences three major physiological changes in her lifetime—the menarche, pregnancy, and the menopause. Over the years pregnancy has unfortunately been medicalised as doctors took over the care of pregnant women, following rigid protocols which prevented choice. This led to a certain amount of dissatisfaction amongst pregnant women at the limitations in choice, lack of control and fragmented care resulting in inconsistencies. The *Changing Childbirth* report[1] advocated increased choices for women, and *First Class Delivery: A National Survey of Women's Views of Maternity Care*[2] reinforced the fact that most women wanted choice, and not the rigidity of the medicalised system.

Women are discouraged from using pharmaceutical preparations during pregnancy because of their potential teratogenic effects on the fetus, and conventional medicine is restricted in what it has to offer expectant mothers for dealing with the discomforts of pregnancy and the pain of labour. The popularity of complementary therapies has increased tremendously in the last 15–20 years, and the use of complementary therapies with midwifery practice is increasing as a result of

---

[1] DEPARTMENT OF HEALTH (1993). *Changing Childbirth: Report of the Expert Maternity Group*. London: HMSO.
[2] AUDIT COMMISSION (1998). *First Class Delivery: A National Survey of Women's Views of Maternity Care*. London: Audit Commission for Local Authorities and the National Health Service in England and Wales.

clients' demands and a desire to be more in control of their own health.

Marion Simpson MEd., Cert Ed., RGN, RM, ADM,
Senior Lecturer Midwifery, School of Human and Health
Sciences, Midwifery Division, University of Huddersfield,
practising aromatherapist, member of ISPA

Note to Readers

Every care has been taken to ensure that the instructions and advice given in this book are accurate and practical. However, where health is concerned—and in particular a serious problem of any kind—it must be stressed that there is no substitute for seeking advice from a qualified medical practitioner. All persistent symptoms, of whatever nature, may have underlying causes that need, and should not be treated without, professional elucidation and evaluation. It is therefore very important, if you intend to use this book for self-help, only to do so in conjunction with duly prescribed conventional or other therapy. In any event, read the advice carefully, and pay particular attention to the precautions and warnings.

The Publisher makes no representation, express or implied, with regard to the accuracy of the information contained in this book, and legal responsibility or liability cannot be accepted by the Author or the Publisher for any errors or omissions that may be made or for any loss, damage, injury or problems suffered or in any way arising from following the advice offered in these pages.

Introduction

Pregnancy is one of the happiest, natural and most exciting times of a woman's life. It is usually also one of the healthiest, when your complexion glows, your hair shines, nails strengthen and you develop that distinctive pregnancy bloom. It is also a time when well-being and relaxation are essential – for the health of both you and your baby.

An alternative – or more accurately, complementary – approach is becoming increasingly popular as pregnancy is a time when drugs are best avoided. Even over-the-counter medicines carry risks and may interfere with the conception and development of your baby. Complementary treatments take an holistic approach and can help you relax to enjoy your pregnancy in the peak of health. And if pregnancy-associated health problems do arise, you will usually find several techniques that can offer a pleasant and rapid solution.

Complementary medicines are powerful tools and need to be treated with respect. In most cases, it is advisable to consult a trained therapist as – just as with certain drugs – some herbs, aromatherapy essential oils, homoeopathic remedies and acupuncture points should be avoided during pregnancy.

There are times when orthodox medicine is needed and you should always follow the advice and treatments recommended by your doctor or obstetrician. Complementary therapies should be just that: techniques to use alongside your medical treatment to complement it where necessary rather than always providing an alternative. Do let your doctor know if you are using a complementary remedy and which ones you have found particularly helpful. The more people inform their doctor about the benefits of holistic therapies, the more doctors will take an interest and start to explore these forms of treatment themselves.

Similarly, do write to me at Souvenir Press, so that I can include your comments (anonymously) as quotes in future editions of this book.

Have a happy and healthy pregnancy. Enjoy.

CHAPTER 1

The Changes of Pregnancy

Pregnancy is a time of great change in which your body adapts to nourish a baby that grows from the size of a microdot to a newborn infant weighing 3 kg or more. Over the nine months of pregnancy, your body undergoes a series of quite profound physical alterations:

- Your need of many vitamins such as folic acid and minerals such as iron and calcium increases.
- Your intestines become more efficient at absorbing a higher percentage of nutrients from your diet.
- Nutrients are better absorbed from your diet as your need for vitamins and minerals increases.
- Your metabolism converts food energy into body fat stores more efficiently so less energy is wasted as heat.
- The way your body handles protein becomes more efficient.
- Your blood sugar level fluctuates as your metabolism adapts to providing enough glucose for you and your growing baby.
- Your womb grows from around the size of a pear to the size of a large beach ball that, towards the end of pregnancy, starts to compress your stomach, bladder, intestines and pelvic veins.
- Your liver and kidneys work harder as they have to process wastes from both you and your growing baby.
- Your breasts enlarge and mature in preparation for milk

1

production. The volume of blood in your circulation increases by a third.

- You build up extra fat reserves to provide energy for breast feeding and you may put on weight in unusual places, such as between your shoulders, on your upper back and around your knees as well as on your hips and thighs.
- You naturally slow down and become less physically active.
- Hormonal levels change considerably and can affect your moods and emotions.
- Your immunity changes so your body does not reject the embryo (fetus), but you become more prone to minor infections such as cystitis and thrush.
- Your temperature regulation may change so that one moment you feel hot and sweaty, and the next cold and clammy. These changes are most common during high summer and deep winter. They seem to be worse at night and during the last ten weeks of pregnancy.

Everyone's metabolism is different, however, and the way pregnancy affects you will be different from the effect it has on your best friend and sometimes even your mother or sister. It all depends on the particular genes you have inherited.

Because of these changes, regular antenatal care is essential to monitor your health throughout the pregnancy, and to ensure your baby is growing and developing normally as nature intended.

Some of the physical changes occurring in the body can result in minor ailments. It is important to keep medications and interventions to a minimum during pregnancy and to take only tablets that are medically essential. Fortunately, many common pregnancy-related conditions can be relieved naturally—either by yourself or through consulting a qualified alternative practitioner. Many complementary therapies are also useful for general relaxation for all pregnant women.

Yoga, meditation, visualisation and massage, for example, are excellent ways to achieve relaxation.

The following pages explore the range of complementary techniques available for use during pregnancy, and the common pregnancy-associated conditions they can help.

CHAPTER 2

Diet and Exercise

A healthy diet and lifestyle can help to overcome many pregnancy-associated conditions and complement a natural approach to health. What you eat and what you do can have a profound effect on your baby's development—especially during the first four weeks after conception—often before you are even aware you are pregnant. Research suggests that the development of coronary heart disease, stroke or diabetes in later life may be linked to poor nutrition in the first few weeks of life when the placenta and the baby's circulation, nervous system and major organs are being laid down. By looking after your diet and lifestyle during pregnancy, you are investing in your baby's future health.

For an optimum healthy diet during pregnancy you need a good intake of each of the following.

Fresh fruit and vegetables: These contain vitamins, minerals, fibre and protective plant substances that may reduce the risk of some cancers. Aim to eat at least five servings of fruit, vegetables and salad stuffs per day, and preferably more. Buy produce as fresh as possible, preferably organic (see p. 11) and use it quickly before its vitamin content decreases. Make sure you wash and, where practical, peel all fruit, salads and vegetables (especially carrots and apples) before eating. Ideally, you need to eat most vegetables apart from potatoes lightly cooked or—if applicable—raw for the greatest nutritional benefit. Where possible, steam for a very short time only. If boiling, bring water to

4

the boil before adding vegetables as this helps to destroy enzymes that break down some vitamins such as vitamin C. The vegetable water can also be used to make sauces, gravy or soup as it is rich in minerals lost from the foods during cooking.

Unrefined complex carbohydrates: Foods such as wholemeal bread, brown rice, wholegrain cereals and wholewheat pasta provide energy, vitamins, trace elements and fibre. They should ideally make up at least half your daily energy intake. Unrefined, complex carbohydrates are also important in helping to maintain stable blood sugar levels during pregnancy, without large swings. The amount that different foods cause blood glucose levels to rise is known as their glycaemic index (GI). For general health—and especially during pregnancy—it is best to eat foods with a low to moderate GI, and to combine foods with a high GI with those that have a lower GI to help even out fluctuations in blood sugar levels. The table on p. 6 shows the glycaemic index of a variety of foods compared with glucose, which has the highest glycaemic index of 100.

Looking at the list, wholemeal pasta is especially good during pregnancy as it falls in the middle GI range. Potatoes, parsnips and carrots have a surprisingly high GI index and are therefore best combined with vegetables of a lower GI such as beans and peas.

Protein-rich foods: These include lean meat, fish, pulses, eggs, milk, cheese, cereals, nuts and seeds. Your need for protein increases by around 15 per cent during pregnancy so it is important to eat a little more of these types of food—especially fish, which is also an important source of healthy fats (see below). Avoid liver and liver products, however, because of the risk of vitamin A toxicity. Vegetarians can obtain protein from pulses, grains, cereals, nuts and seeds.

Glycaemic index values of some common foods

FOOD	GI	FOOD	GI
Glucose	100	Ice-cream	50–61
Baked potatoes	98	Cake	50
Parsnips	97	Carrots	49
Brown rice	82	Chocolate bar	49
Cornflakes	80	Grapes	44
Weetabix	75	Wholemeal pasta	42
Wholemeal bread	72	Peaches	42
Shredded Wheat	67	Baked beans	40
Raisins	64	Oranges	40
Bananas	62	Apples	39
Chocolate biscuit	59	Milk (skimmed)	32
Porridge oats	54	Kidney beans	29
Crisps	51	Grapefruit	26

Foods rich in healthy fats: These include oily fish, nuts and seeds including olive oil, rapeseed oil, walnut oil and evening primrose oil. While most people need to eat less fat overall, it is important whilst pregnant to increase the proportion of the healthy fats in your diet. Oily fish (e.g. sardines, salmon, herring, mackerel) contain essential fatty acids (EFAs), which are beneficial for your circulation, and which are also important for the development of your baby's brain, nervous system and eyes. EFAs help to protect against the chance of your baby developing dyslexia, attention deficit hyperactivity disorder, autism or possibly even schizophrenia in future life. They are also converted into hormone-like chemicals called prostaglandins, which help to ensure the healthy development of your baby, reduce the risk of premature delivery, protect against high blood pressure during pregnancy and soften your cervix to trigger childbirth when the time is right. A good intake of EFAs may also help to prevent the lack of concentration, poor memory, forgetfulness and vagueness that many women experience during the last few months of pregnancy. Anecdotal evidence also suggests that taking evening primrose oil supplements may help to prevent stretch marks by improving the suppleness and quality of your skin.

A healthy adult woman needs around 6–10 g EFAs per day. During pregnancy and breast feeding, these needs are increased to an average of 14 g EFAs per day. Unfortunately, eight out of ten pregnant women have too low an intake of EFAs. Ideally you need to eat oily fish *at least* two or three times per week. If you don't like fish, supplements containing fish oils and evening primrose oil are available especially designed to be taken during pregnancy and breast feeding.

NB: Do not take products containing cod liver oil during pregnancy as this contains vitamin A, an excess of which can be harmful to a developing baby.

Interestingly, studies suggest that if you are carrying a male baby you need a higher intake of EFAs than if you are carrying a female baby. Consider taking evening primrose oil (500 mg to 1 g per day). New essential fatty acid supplements especially designed for pregnancy are now also available. These include evening primrose oil and/or essential fatty acids derived from fish oils (e.g. Efanatal), from microalgae (e.g. Neuromins, available in the US) or tuna oil (Milkarra). These may be taken when planning a pregnancy, whilst expecting and when breast feeding.

Lack of essential fatty acids can cause symptoms including:

- itchy skin;
- thirst;
- urinary frequency;
- dry, rough, pimply skin;
- itchy skin;
- dry hair;
- dandruff;
- brittle nails;
- lowered immunity with frequent infections.

NB: If you develop severe itching, thirst or urinary symptoms during pregnancy, you should always seek medical advice as these symptoms can also be due to other problems needing different treatment.

An optimum intake of EFAs during pregnancy can:

- improve the development of your baby's eyes and visual acuity;
- improve your baby's brain and optimise intelligence;
- reduce your risk of a preterm delivery or a low birth weight baby;
- reduce your risk of pregnancy-associated high blood pressure (pre-eclampsia);
- reduce your risk of poor concentration and forgetfulness during pregnancy;
- reduce your risk of dry, itchy skin problems and possibly stretch marks.

ENERGY INTAKE

You need an extra 70 000 kcal during pregnancy—both for the development of your baby and to lay down body fat stores needed for breast feeding. You don't need to eat for two, however. Your metabolism will automatically become more efficient so that more of your energy intake is made use of rather than wasted as heat. You will also naturally cut down your level of activity as pregnancy progresses so you use up less energy through exercise. In fact, you do not need to increase your calorie intake during the first six months of pregnancy. During the last three months you need an extra 200 kcal per day and when breast feeding you will need 450–570 kcal more per day than before you were pregnant. It is important not to overeat, however, as you will then put on excess weight, which may cause problems in later pregnancy and be difficult to lose afterwards. Ideally, a normal weight woman needs to gain between 11.5 kg (25 lb) and 16 kg (35 lb) to allow her baby to grow properly. Even women who are obese need to gain between 7 kg (9 lb) and 11.5 kg (25 lb) during pregnancy, while those who are underweight should try to gain between 12.5 kg and 18 kg. The average weight gain during 40 weeks pregnancy is around 12.5 kg (27.6 lb).

Average increase in weight (g) during pregnancy and where it goes

	10 WEEKS	20 WEEKS	30 WEEKS	40 WEEKS
Your baby	5	300	1500	3300
The placenta	20	170	430	650

	10 WEEKS	20 WEEKS	30 WEEKS	40 WEEKS
Amniotic fluid	30	250	600	800
Uterus	135	585	810	900
Breasts	35	180	360	400
Extra blood	100	600	1300	1200
Extra fat/fluid	325	1915	3500	5200
Total weight gain	650	4000	8500	12 500

FOODS RICH IN FOLIC ACID

Increase your intake of foods rich in folic acid as these can help reduce the risk of some developmental defects, including spina bifida. Good dietary sources of folic acid include green leafy vegetables (e.g. spinach, broccoli, Brussels sprouts, kale and spring greens), pulses and foods fortified with folic acid (e.g. some breakfast cereals). Manufacturers have also started putting a blue flash on packets to make it easier to select foods fortified with folic acid; these include cereals and some bread (see p. 24).

FOODS RICH IN IRON

Vegetarian mothers-to-be need to pay special attention to their dietary intake of iron (see p. 32). The form of iron that is most easily absorbed is organic haem iron, which is found in red meat. Vegetarians, and those who eat little red meat, are therefore at increased risk of iron deficiency. Their intakes are dependent on absorbing inorganic non-haem iron, and food supplements are essential.

GOING ORGANIC

Consider following an organic diet during pregnancy. The full effects of agricultural chemicals (e.g. pesticides, weedkillers, fungicides, fumigants, growth promoters, growth retardants and fertilisers) on fertility and reproductive health are still not fully understood. Apart from anything else, research shows that organic foods contain, on average, twice the nutrient content of commercially grown produce. This is partly because they contain less water and more solid matter, but also because of the naturally enriched soils in which they are grown.

A HEALTHY DIET DURING PREGNANCY

When you are pregnant, aim to:

- eat a good, healthy, varied diet;
- eat according to your appetite;
- if you are hungry, have a healthy snack such as fruit, toast, bread, plain biscuits, malt loaf, yoghurt or fromage frais; aim to eat three meals and three snacks per day during the last six months of pregnancy;
- take a vitamin and mineral supplement especially formulated for pregnancy;
- drink plenty of fluids but avoid alcohol as much as possible (see p. 13).

Eat more:

- fruit or vegetables—at least five portions per day;
- vegetarian meals;
- lean white meat e.g. chicken;
- oily fish or take a fish oil supplement;
- bread, pasta, rice and plain potatoes;
- pulses, nuts and seeds;

- grilled, steamed, poached or casseroled food;
- baked potatoes;
- foods fortified with folic acid;
- mineral water or fruit/herbal teas.

Cut down on your intake of:

- foods of little nutritional value e.g. biscuits, cakes, confectionery, crisps, pastries and fizzy drinks;
- highly processed foods full of additives;
- refined (table) sugar;
- salt;
- fatty foods e.g. doughnuts, fatty meat, cream, roast or fried foods such as chips.

REDUCING THE RISK OF FOOD POISONING

Pregnant women are particularly susceptible to some food-borne infections owing to their altered immunity, and because infections that may prove harmless to the mother can seriously affect the baby's development. Keep your kitchen clean and dry and, as part of normal hygiene practice, wash your hands thoroughly before preparing foods. It is also a good idea to keep pets out of the kitchen at all times. Store raw meat at the bottom of the fridge, covered, and separate from cooked foods. To reduce the risk of infection, the temperature of your fridge should be below 5 °C and that of your freezer below minus 18 °C. Frozen produce must be defrosted thoroughly before cooking and all foods should be cooked or reheated thoroughly. Throw away all foods past their 'best by' date.

Avoid foods that can increase the risk of infection with *Salmonella*, *Listeria* or *Toxoplasma* such as:

- ripened soft cheeses e.g. Brie, Camembert and Cambozola;
- blue-veined cheeses e.g. Stilton, Roquefort, Blue Shropshire, Blue Brie and Dolcelatte;

- goat or sheep cheeses e.g. feta and Chèvre;
- any unpasteurised soft and cream cheese
  (**NB: All hard Cheddar-type cheeses are safe, as are cottage cheese, soft processed cheese spreads and cream cheese**);
- any undercooked (raw, rare or pink) meat;
- raw eggs or any that are not fully hard boiled;
- cook–chill meals and ready-to-eat poultry unless thoroughly reheated;
- all types of pâté;
- ready-prepared coleslaw and salads;
- unwrapped foods that are not reheated thoroughly (e.g. sausage rolls);
- unpasteurised milk or dairy products;
- shellfish;
- rolls or sandwiches containing any of the above;
- soft whipped ice-cream from ice-cream machines.

ALCOHOL

Try to avoid alcohol altogether during the three months before trying to conceive, and throughout pregnancy if you can. Alcohol is a cell poison that becomes concentrated in the cells of a developing baby to produce higher levels than in the mother. Avoiding even small amounts of alcohol can reduce the risk of miscarriage, and congenital defects.

Some studies suggest that low intakes of alcohol (up to eight units in a week) are not harmful during later pregnancy but the best advice is to avoid alcohol altogether for at least the first three months of pregnancy. If you find it difficult to go without alcohol after this, the odd drink (one or two units) once or twice a week during the later stages of pregnancy is unlikely to cause serious harm but may increase the risk of miscarriage.

1 unit alcohol   = 100 ml (one glass) of wine
               = 50 ml (one measure) of sherry
               = 25 ml (single tot) of spirit
               = 300 ml (½ pint) of normal strength
                  beer.

VITAMINS AND MINERALS

During pregnancy your need for certain vitamins and minerals increases and over half the nutrients you eat are used by your growing baby—one of many reasons why you may feel tired even during the early months while your baby is still quite tiny. Studies show that a good maternal diet around the time of conception and during pregnancy significantly reduces the risk of having a baby with a low birth weight, which is one of the commonest causes of serious health problems in the newborn. Healthy diet is especially important when you have a multiple pregnancy as you have to nourish two or more infants rather than one. At present, the only supplement universally recommended when planning a baby and during pregnancy is folic acid, which can reduce the risk of certain congenital problems (neural tube defects) such as spina bifida by 75 per cent. Other nutrients such as B12 and certain trace minerals can reduce this risk even further, however. In fact, taking a multivitamin supplement for at least one month before conception and for at least two months after has been shown to reduce the risk of all major congenital abnormalities by at least half, while the risks of some problems such as urinary tract abnormalities may be reduced by as much as 85 per cent.

Unfortunately, women of childbearing age in the Western world are likely to have intakes below the recommended daily amount (RDA) for a wide range of nutrients, including folic acid, vitamins A, B6, C, E, iron and zinc. Studies have also found that intakes of calcium and magnesium in pregnant

14

Taking a multivitamin and mineral supplement has been shown to reduce the risk of:

- all congenital developmental defects in general;
- urinary tract abnormalities by 85 per cent;
- neural tube defects by at least 50 per cent;
- facial abnormality, cleft lip or cleft palate by 25–50 per cent;
- some limb abnormalities by 35 per cent;
- heart defects by 35 per cent;
- low birth weight;
- maternal night cramps during pregnancy.

---

women are frequently below the RDA, although the significance of this is still uncertain.

Whilst it is important to obtain vitamins and minerals in adequate amounts, it is also important not to take too much as some can be harmful in excess. Although diet should always come first, it is a good idea to take a vitamin and mineral supplement especially designed for pregnancy. Several different brands are available, and your pharmacist can advise on which would suit you best.

The following table shows the new EU RDA for adults, the UK reference nutrient intakes (RNI) from women aged 19–50 years, together with the government reference nutrient intakes (RNIs) recommended for pregnant women. The RNIs drawn up in 1991 accept that pregnant women need more vitamin A, thiamin (vitamin B1), riboflavin (vitamin B2), vitamin C, vitamin D and folic acid than do non-pregnant women, but surprisingly claim that a woman needs no other vitamins or additional minerals during pregnancy. This seems strange as, in many cases, the recommended intakes for UK pregnant women are less than the EU RDAs for non-pregnant adult women. These recommendations need urgent updating, not just for the health of mother and baby during pregnancy, but for the long-term health of the mother's bones and her future risk of osteoporosis.

Recommended daily intakes for adult women

NUTRIENT	NON-PREGNANT		PREGNANT	BREAST-FEEDING
	EU RDA	RNI women (19–50 years)	RNI	RNI
Vitamin A (retinol)	800 mcg	600 mcg	+100 mcg	+350 mcg
Vitamin B1 (thiamin)	1.4 mg	0.8 mg	+0.1 mg	+0.2 mg
Vitamin B2 (riboflavin)	1.6 mg	1.1 mg	+0.3 mg	+0.5 mg
Vitamin B3 (niacin)	18 mg	13 mg	—	+2 mg
Vitamin B5 (pantothenic acid)	6 mg	not set		
Vitamin B6 (pyridoxine)	2 mg	1.2 mg	—	—
Vitamin B12 (cyanocobalamin)	1 mcg	1.5 mcg	—	+0.5 mcg
Folate	200 mcg	200 mcg	400 mcg*	+60 mcg
Biotin	150 mcg	not set		
Vitamin C	60 mg	40 mg	+10 mg	+30 mg
Vitamin D	5 mcg	**	10 mcg	10 mcg
Vitamin E	10 mg	not set		
Calcium	800 mg	700 mg	—	+550 mg

NUTRIENT	NON-PREGNANT		PREGNANT	BREAST-FEEDING
	EU RDA	RNI women (19–50 years)	RNI	RNI
Copper	1.1 mg	1.2 mg	—	+0.3 mg
Iodine	150 mcg	140 mcg	—	—
Iron	14 mg	14.8 mg	—	—
Magnesium	300 mg	270 mg	—	+50 mg
Phosphorus	800 mg	550 mg	—	+440 mg
Selenium	not set	60 mcg	—	+15 mcg
Zinc	15 mg	7 mg	—	+6 mg 0–4 months; +2.5 mg thereafter assuming your baby has started to wean

EU RDA = EU recommended daily amount; RNI = UK reference nutrient intake; mg = milligrams; mcg = micrograms (i.e. 10^{-6} grams).

(—) No increase suggested.

(*) Plus increased intake of folate-rich food during preconceptual period until at least 12 weeks of pregnancy. Women who have previously had a child with a neural tube defect need increased intake of folate-rich foods plus 4 mg (4000 mcg) folate during the preconceptual care period until at least the 12th week of pregnancy.

(**) No RNI needed for people who receive exposure to sunlight. An RNI of 10 mcg is suggested for those confined indoors.

Minerals

Some researchers have suggested that women need the following additional minerals during pregnancy.

MINERAL	ADDITIONAL REQUIREMENTS SUGGESTED FOR PREGNANCY
Calcium	an extra 300 mg per day
Chromium III	an extra 100 mcg per day
Copper	an extra 0.5 mg per day
Iron	an extra 10 mg per day
Magnesium	an extra 100 mg per day
Zinc	an extra 10 mg per day

Vitamins

Vitamin A (retinol)

This vitamin helps to control the growth and development of your baby by regulating genes needed to produce some proteins, including enzymes. It also has an important role as an antioxidant and may provide some protection against cerebral palsy. While it is essential, excess vitamin A is toxic during pregnancy at just three times the normal recommended daily intake for adults. Intakes of more than 10 000 international units (IU) of vitamin A supplements, for example, increase the risk of a developmental abnormality affecting the head, brain or spinal cord by a factor of five. The most harmful time to take excess vitamin A seems to be the first seven weeks of pregnancy. Some experts therefore advise against taking supplements containing preformed vitamin A (retinol) unless prescribed by a doctor to treat proven low levels. Others feel that supplements containing vitamin A may be safely used by pregnant women who follow standard advice to consume little or no liver or liver products, which have a naturally high vitamin A content.

Always avoid cod liver oil supplements, liver and liver products during pregnancy. The safest way to take vitamin A is as betacarotene—a yellow vegetable pigment that consists of two vitamin A molecules joined together. When vitamin A is

18

needed, the betacarotene is broken down to top up supplies.

How much you need: The UK reference nutrient intake for vitamin A is 700 mcg (micrograms) per day. World Health Organisation (WHO) recommendations are higher, at 800 mcg vitamin A daily for adult women and 1000 mcg per day during pregnancy. Most pregnant women in the western world already have a vitamin A intake greater than this, although deficiency is a common problem in underdeveloped countries.

Good dietary sources of vitamin A for pregnant women include:

- meat;
- eggs;
- milk, butter, cheese and yoghurt;
- oily fish;
- margarine.

Good dietary sources of betacarotene include:

- dark green leafy vegetables e.g. spinach, broccoli and spring greens;
- yellow-orange vegetables and fruits e.g. carrots, sweet potatoes, cantaloupe melons, apricots, peaches, mangoes, red-yellow peppers and sweet corn.

Vitamin B1 (thiamin)
This is needed for the production of energy, manufacture of red blood cells and the synthesis of some amino acids. It is essential for normal growth and development of your baby, especially the brain and nervous system. If your diet is lacking in thiamin, you have a higher risk of a low birth weight baby.

How much you need: The EU RDA for adults is 1.4 mg (milligrams) daily. The UK recommendation is 0.8 mg per day for women, with an additional 0.1 mg during the last three months of pregnancy (0.9 mg).

Good dietary sources for pregnant women include:

- brewer's yeast and yeast extracts;
- brown rice;
- wholegrain cereals, wheatgerm, wholewheat pasta, oatmeal and oatflakes;
- soya and other pulses;
- meat;
- seafood;
- nuts.

Vitamin B2 (riboflavin)

This is needed for good immunity, the production of energy and for the metabolism of proteins, fats and carbohydrate. It is also an important antioxidant. Vitamin B2 is so important for a baby's growth that 15 to 30 per cent of your B2 intake will enter your breast milk to nourish your newborn baby.

How much you need: The US recommendation for pregnant women and nursing mothers is 2–2.5 mg per day. The EU RDA for adults is 1.6 mg, while the UK RNI for riboflavin is 1.4 mg per day during pregnancy and 1.6 mg during lactation.

Good dietary sources for pregnant women include:

- yeast extract;
- wholegrain cereals, wheatgerm and bran;
- eggs;
- milk, cheese, yoghurt;
- green leafy vegetables;
- beans.

Vitamin B3 (niacin)

This is essential for releasing energy from body stores and for the handling of oxygen in rapidly dividing cells such as those of your developing baby, as rapidly dividing cells use a lot of oxygen in cell respiration. It is also important for healthy skin, nerves and brain cells. Niacin also works together with mineral chromium to control the way cells take up glucose. Lack of niacin (or chromium) may increase your chance of developing diabetes in pregnancy.

How much you need: The National Research Council in America recommends an adult daily intake of 13–19 mg per day. The EU RDA is 18 mg niacin for adults. In the UK, 13 mg per day is suggested for both pregnant and non-pregnant women, with an additional 2 mg per day when breast feeding.

Good dietary sources for pregnant women include:

- yeast extract;
- wholegrains, brown rice and wheatbran;
- nuts and dried fruit;
- meat and poultry;
- oily fish;
- eggs;
- milk and cheese.

Vitamin B5 (pantothenic acid)
This is needed to metabolise proteins, fat and carbohydrates, for making some adrenal hormones and for a healthy nervous system.

How much you need: The EU RDA for adults is 6 mg per day.

Good dietary sources for pregnant women include:

- yeast extract;
- wholegrains, wheatgerm and bran;
- meat and poultry;
- eggs;
- beans, nuts and vegetables.

21

Vitamin B6 (pyridoxine)
This is involved in the action of over 60 metabolic enzymes including those needed to make genetic material, antibodies, proteins for metabolising body stores of carbohydrate and essential fatty acids. It is especially important during rapid cell division such as that occurring during pregnancy. It also helps to regulate the sex hormones.

How much you need: The US and EU RDAs for vitamin B6 are 2 mg for adults, while the UK reference nutrient intake is lower at 1.2 mg per day for both non-pregnant and pregnant women.

Good dietary sources for pregnant women include:

- yeast extract;
- wholegrain cereals and brown rice;
- meat;
- oily fish;
- soya products;
- bananas, walnuts and avocado;
- green leafy vegetables.

Excessively large doses of vitamin B6 during pregnancy may increase the risk of congenital limb abnormalities in the offspring so do not take very high dose supplements.

Vitamin B12 (cobalamin)
This is needed, together with folic acid, for making new copies of genetic material when cells divide. Lack of either vitamin leads to abnormally large cells that can lead to anaemia and increase the risk of certain developmental disorders. Lack of vitamin B12 now seems to be an independent risk factor for neural tube defects, which are five times more common in babies whose mothers have low blood levels of vitamin B12, whether or not folic acid levels are low. Some researchers now suggest that B12 supplements should be included in pro-

grammes designed to reduce the risk of neural tube defects. New research also suggests that lack of vitamin B12 may be linked with an increased risk of having a baby with autism.

How much you need: The EU RDA and UK RNI for vitamin B12 is 1.5 mcg per day. No additional supplements are yet suggested during pregnancy, although an extra 0.5 mcg per day is needed whilst breast feeding. Some countries recommend an adult intake of 3 mcg per day.

Good dietary sources for pregnant women include:

● yeast extracts;
● fish—especially sardines;
● red meat;
● eggs;
● milk, cheese and yoghurt.

Folic acid (folate)
This is the only vitamin that you require double the amount of during pregnancy than at other times and it can take more than six months after childbirth for your folic acid needs to return to normal levels. Folic acid is needed for copying genetic material and the healthy division of cells, for healthy nerves and for the metabolism of sugars and proteins. If folate is lacking, dividing cells become abnormally large and are more likely to contain abnormal chromosomes.

Lack of folic acid during the first few weeks of pregnancy, when the brain and spinal cord are being laid down, is associated with a form of congenital abnormality known as a neural tube defect (e.g. spina bifida), and with an increased risk of cleft palate, hare lip and abnormalities of the limbs, heart, lungs and skeleton. Sadly, at least two babies are conceived with a neural tube defect in the UK every day. It is now suggested that every woman of childbearing age should take supplements containing 400 mcg folic acid. This is especially important when planning to conceive and for at least the first 12 weeks of pregnancy. If a woman who has previously had a child with a neural tube defect takes 4 mg folic acid daily from before conception until the 12th week of gestation, her risk of a recurrence is reduced by 70 per cent compared with similar women who took no folic acid supplements or other vitamins. Similarly, women taking multivitamins including folic acid throughout the first six weeks of gestation had around 70 per cent fewer affected pregnancies compared with those who took multivitamins without folic acid.

If you have epilepsy, and are taking drugs to stop your seizures, you should seek medical advice before trying for a baby. Some anticonvulsant drugs work by interfering with the way your body handles folic acid, so supplements can affect your treatment. It is best to seek specialist advice about which antiepilepsy drugs are safe to take during pregnancy (you may need your medication changed), and what level of folic acid supplementation you need.

How much you need: Increase your intake of folic acid in three ways as follows:

- Take a supplement providing 400 mcg folic acid daily. If you have previously conceived a child with a neural tube defect, you should take a supplement containing at least ten times more folic acid. Supplements containing 5 mg folic acid are available on prescription for this purpose.
- Choose foods that have been fortified with folic acid; these include many breakfast cereals and some breads. They are now easier to spot thanks to the Health Education Authority's (HEA's) 'flash' scheme, which leading manufacturers are adding to their packaging. Look out for flashes saying: 'contains folic acid'—on foods that can provide at least one-sixth of your daily requirement—and 'with extra folic acid'—on foods enriched to provide at least half your daily requirements.

- Eat more foods that are naturally rich in folic acid (see below).

You should start increasing your folic acid intake from the time you first start trying to conceive, and for at least the first 12 weeks of pregnancy and preferably throughout the whole nine months.

Good dietary sources for pregnant women include:

- fortified foods;
- yeast extract;
- green leafy vegetables e.g. spinach, broccoli, Brussels sprouts, kale and spring greens;
- soya beans, green beans, chickpeas, cooked black-eye beans and baked beans;
- wholemeal or granary-style bread;
- asparagus, avocados and cauliflowers;
- milk, butter, cheese, cottage cheese and yoghurt;
- eggs.

Biotin

Biotin is needed for the metabolism of glucose and important fatty acids, proteins and genetic building blocks whose synthesis increases during pregnancy. Biotin is so important for your baby's growth and development that it also becomes concentrated in your breast milk to 15 times the level found in your bloodstream. Lack of biotin has been linked with severe cradle-cap in newborn babies.

How much you need: The US recommended daily amount for biotin is 300 mcg per day. The EU RDA for adults is 150 mcg (0.15 mg).

Good dietary sources for pregnant women are:

- yeast extract;
- wholegrain cereals, rice and wholemeal bread;

- nuts and seeds;
- oily fish, especially sardines;
- egg yolks.

Vitamin C

This is essential for making collagen—an important protein found in just about every part of your growing baby. It is needed for proper growth and repair and for healthy skin, bones, teeth and hormone balance. It also acts as a powerful antioxidant that helps to protect against genetic damage and may provide some protection against cerebral palsy. Vitamin C is so important for your baby's well-being that its vitamin C levels in the womb are 10 per cent higher than your own. Some evidence suggests that taking vitamin C supplements during pregnancy may halve the risk of offspring developing a childhood tumour. Lack of vitamin C has also been linked with an increased risk of premature rupture of membranes and preterm labour as a result of producing poor quality collagen that breaks down more easily.

When maternal intakes of vitamin C were assessed during breast feeding, it was found that those with low intakes during the last three months of pregnancy had significantly lower levels of vitamin C in breast milk. It is important that women increase their intake of vitamin C during pregnancy by eating more fruits and vegetables.

How much you need: The US and EU RDA is 60 mg per day for adults. In the US, pregnant women are advised to obtain 70 mg vitamin C daily, increasing to 95 mg per day when breast feeding. Some researchers now believe that supplements containing at least 250 mg vitamin C may be a good idea during pregnancy and breast feeding.

Good dietary sources for pregnant women include:

- berry fruits (e.g. blackcurrants, strawberries and black-berries);
- citrus fruit;
- kiwi fruit;
- mangoes, guavas;
- capsicum peppers;
- green leafy vegetables e.g. broccoli, Brussels sprouts, watercress and parsley.

Vitamin D

Vitamin D is both a vitamin and a hormone. It is needed to absorb calcium and phosphate from the diet and is essential for the formation of healthy bones and teeth. It can be made in the body by the action of sunlight on your skin, but dietary sources are also very important—especially during winter.

How much you need: The EU RDA for vitamin D is 10 mcg per day.

Good dietary source for pregnant women include:

- oily fish e.g. sardines, herrings, mackerel, salmon and trout;
- butter and fortified margarine;
- fortified milk;
- eggs.

Excess vitamin D (above 250 mg per day) is toxic, however, so avoid megadoses.

Vitamin E

This is a powerful antioxidant that protects body fats, cell membranes, nerves and brain tissues from damaging chemical reactions known as oxidation. It also helps to strengthen muscle fibres, including those in your developing baby's heart, and may reduce the risk of miscarriage as well as making childbirth easier. Vitamin E at high doses (300 mg daily)

27

seemed to reduce the risk of complications associated with uterine fibroids during pregnancy. A good intake of vitamin E during pregnancy may help to protect against cerebral palsy and more than halve the risk of offspring developing a childhood brain tumour. Vitamin E also helps to keep skin healthy and may reduce the risk of stretch marks. Premature infants often have low levels of vitamin E, which makes their red blood cell membranes fragile and may contribute to neonatal anaemia and jaundice.

How much you need: The EU RDA is 10 mg per day. Many experts now believe that higher intakes are needed for optimum antioxidant protection. Taking extra vitamin E during pregnancy (e.g. 67 mg, equivalent to 100 IU) seems reasonable. Supplements should ideally be vitamin E (D-α-tocopherol) from a natural source and not synthetic DL-α-tocopherol, which is less active.

Good dietary sources for pregnant women include:

- vegetable oils, of which wheatgerm oil is the richest;
- avocados, pears;
- wholegrain cereals and wholemeal bread;
- butter and margarine;
- eggs;
- nuts and seeds;
- oily fish;
- dark green leafy vegetables (e.g. broccoli).

Minerals

Calcium
Calcium is important during pregnancy for developing healthy bones, muscle contraction and the transmission of nerve signals. It is the only mineral whose requirement *doubles* during pregnancy; if your diet is poor in calcium, it will be leached

from your own stores—your bones and teeth. A good intake is therefore important to prevent pregnancy-associated osteoporosis (see p. 192). Research also suggests that a good intake of calcium (including supplements) can more than halve the risk of developing pregnancy-associated high blood pressure (pre-eclampsia) and, furthermore, can lower high blood pressure in women who develop this condition. Importantly, babies born to mothers with a poor calcium intake tend to have a low birth weight and slow development.

How much you need: The EU RDA and UK RNI for calcium is 800 mg per day; surprisingly no extra is recommended during pregnancy, although an extra 550 mg per day is suggested when breast feeding. Some research suggests the optimal intake of calcium during pregnancy and breast feeding is 1200–1500 mg per day. The National Osteoporosis Society recommend the following calcium intakes for women:

- non-pregnant women 19–44 years   1000 mg calcium per day
- pregnant women   1200 mg calcium per day
- breast-feeding mothers   1250 mg per day

Interestingly, calcium absorption from the gut seems to be more efficient during pregnancy. This is secondary to a natural increase in blood levels of vitamin D—without any obvious increase in intake or increased exposure to the sun.

Good dietary sources for pregnant women include:

- milk, cheese, yoghurt and fromage frais;
- green leafy vegetables e.g. broccoli;
- salmon;
- pulses, nuts and seeds;
- white and brown bread, both of which are fortified with calcium in the UK;

- oranges;
- eggs.

The easiest way to increase your calcium intake during pregnancy is to drink an extra pint of skimmed or semi-skimmed milk per day. This provides as much calcium as whole milk, but without the additional saturated fat.

Chromium

Chromium forms a complex together with vitamin B3 (niacin) and three amino acids, known as a glucose tolerance factor (GTF). This helps to control blood sugar levels, and adequate intakes of chromium are thought to be important in helping to protect against gestational diabetes.

How much you need: The National Research Council in the US suggests 50–200 mcg per day for an adult. Average intakes are below 50 mcg and deficiency is common, especially among pregnant women.

Good dietary sources for pregnant women include:

- brewer's yeast—the chromium in which is already in the form of GTF and is 50 times more effective than other sources;
- egg yolks;
- red meat;
- cheese;
- fruit, vegetables and juices;
- wholegrain cereals;
- honey;
- black pepper.

Copper

Copper is needed for healthy brain function, healthy bones, cartilage, hair and skin and for production of haemoglobin (the red blood pigment that carries oxygen round the body—see below).

How much you need: The UK RNI is 1.2 mg copper. An extra 0.3 mg is recommended when breast feeding, and some experts suggest an extra 0.5 mg during pregnancy as well. Copper and zinc interfere with one another and, in general, you need a zinc to copper intake ratio of 10 zinc : 1 copper so an intake of around 15 mg zinc and 1.5 mg copper is ideal. Excess copper is toxic.

Good dietary sources for pregnant women include:

- crustaceans e.g. prawns;
- brewer's yeast;
- olives, nuts and pulses;
- wholegrain cereals;
- green vegetables.

Iodine

Iodine is essential for making thyroid hormones; iodine deficiency during pregnancy can lead to an underactive thyroid, which shows up after birth as a condition known as cretinism in which the brain does not develop properly. Lack of iodine is a serious problem in some parts of the world, including parts of Europe, New Zealand, Brazil, Indonesia and the Himalayas. This devastating condition can be prevented by giving iodine supplements to mothers at risk—preferably before becoming pregnant or before they are six months pregnant if treatment is to be successful. In the West, newborn babies are screened for cretinism as part of the heel-prick test carried out soon after birth.

How much you need: The EU RDA is 150 mcg and the UK RNI 140 mcg with no extra suggested for pregnancy. In the US, 150 mcg is recommended for adults, increasing to 175 mcg per day during pregnancy.

Good dietary sources for pregnant women include:

- seafood e.g. haddock, halibut, salmon, tuna, prawns and lobster;

- seaweed (e.g. kelp);
- iodised salt;
- milk, cheese, butter, yoghurt and fromage frais (as cattle feed is also iodised).

Iron

Iron forms part of the red blood pigment, haemoglobin, which carries oxygen around both your body and that of your baby. It is also involved in the production of energy and in immunity. Women suffering from iron deficiency in pregnancy are much more likely to develop candida (thrush) infections, for example. You need more iron during pregnancy as your total blood volume increases by around a third. A common symptom of lack of iron during pregnancy is a craving for strange foods such as soil or coal; this is known as pica. If it happens to you during pregnancy, start taking a supplement containing iron immediately—ask your pharmacist or doctor for advice on dosage. Your doctor may also want to perform a blood test to check your iron stores as iron deficiency increases the risk of poor fetal growth and low birth weight.

How much you need: US recommended dietary allowances suggest that iron requirements should double during pregnancy, from 15 mg to 30 mg per day. The EU RDA for adults is 14 mg, while the UK reference nutrient intake is 14.8 mg per day. The UK does not suggest any additional iron during pregnancy unless a woman has previously had heavy periods (putting her at risk of iron deficiency anaemia). Lack of dietary iron is common, however, and intakes are frequently 30 per cent lower than recommended. A supplement specially formulated for pregnancy that contains some iron is therefore a good idea.

Avoid taking too much iron as this can cause constipation or indigestion, and excess is toxic. Iron supplements given alone can decrease the absorption of zinc, as well as other essential minerals (e.g. manganese, chromium and selenium) so some specialists advise that iron should be given in combination with these.

Good dietary sources for pregnant women include:

- red meat;
- seafood, especially sardines;
- brewer's yeast;
- wholegrain cereals and wheatgerm;
- egg yolks;
- green leafy vegetables;
- dried fruit e.g. prunes.

Haem iron found in red meat is most easily absorbed. Vegetarians, and those who eat little red meat, are therefore at increased risk of iron deficiency. Overboiling vegetables decreases their iron availability by up to 20 per cent. Vitamin C increases the absorption of inorganic iron, whilst calcium and tannin-containing drinks (e.g. tea) decrease it. Wash iron tablets down with orange juice rather than coffee, as coffee can reduce iron absorption by up to 39 per cent if drunk within an hour of eating. Your absorption of dietary iron generally becomes more efficient during pregnancy, however.

Magnesium

Magnesium is needed for every major metabolic reaction in your body, from the synthesis of protein and genetic material to the production of energy. It is therefore essential for healthy development of your baby. Average intakes are low and deficiency may increase the risk of miscarriage, premature delivery and painful contractions during childbirth.

How much you need: The EU RDA for adults is 300 mg. The UK RNI for adult women is 270 mg per day. No increment is suggested during pregnancy, although an extra 50 mg is recommended during lactation. In the US, a daily intake of

280 mg magnesium is recommended for women, with an additional 40 mg per day during pregnancy and an extra 60–75 mg daily during breast feeding.

Good dietary sources for pregnant women include:

- soya beans;
- brewer's yeast;
- wholegrain cereals and brown rice;
- seafood;
- meat;
- eggs;
- milk, cheese, butter, yoghurt and fromage frais;
- bananas, nuts and seeds;
- dark green leafy vegetables.

Manganese
Manganese is essential for normal growth, development and brain function. It is involved in many metabolic reactions, including the production of proteins, carbohydrates and some pregnancy hormones.

How much you need: The optimal intake of manganese is unknown and there is no UK reference nutrient intake. In the US, a daily intake of 2–5 mg is considered adequate, while up to 10 mg per day is thought to be safe.

Good dietary sources for pregnant women include:

- tea;
- wholegrain cereals;
- nuts and seeds;
- fruit;
- eggs;
- green leafy vegetables or herbs;
- milk, cheese, butter, yoghurt and fromage frais.

Selenium

Selenium is vital for growth and immunity, including antibody production. It is also an important antioxidant. Selenium levels fall during pregnancy, and maintaining good levels may decrease the risk of miscarriage, congenital defects and even sudden infant death syndrome.

How much you need: There is no EU RDA for selenium. The UK RNI is 60 mcg with an additional 15 mcg suggested during breast feeding. Selenium intakes in the UK have halved over the last 20 years, to less than 40 mcg per day.

Good dietary sources for pregnant women include:

- broccoli and cabbage;
- mushrooms, radishes and celery;
- onions and garlic;
- wholegrain cereals;
- nuts and seeds;
- brewer's yeast;
- seafood;
- butter;
- vegetables grown in selenium-rich soil.

Zinc

Zinc is essential for over a hundred different enzymes to work properly, including those involved in reading genetic information during fetal growth and development. It also has an antioxidant role. Many pregnant women have low dietary intakes of zinc, and maternal blood zinc levels fall by around 30 per cent during pregnancy, although those of the developing baby are usually double the maternal levels. Adequate intakes of zinc during pregnancy help to protect against low birth weight, miscarriage, pre-eclampsia, anaemia, preterm delivery and some congenital defects. Good levels are also needed for efficient contractions during labour.

How much you need: The EU RDA is 15 mg per day for adults. The UK RNI is only 7 mg, but an extra 6 mg is recommended during pregnancy and 2.5 mg when breast feeding. In the US a daily intake of 12 mg zinc is recommended for non-pregnant women, 15 mg per day during pregnancy and up to 19 mg per day during lactation.

One of the earliest symptoms of zinc deficiency is loss of taste sensation. This can be tested for by obtaining a solution of zinc sulphate (5 mg per 5 ml) from a chemist. Swirl a teaspoonful of the solution in your mouth. If it seems tasteless then zinc deficiency is likely. If the solution tastes furry, of minerals or slightly sweet, your zinc levels are borderline. If it tastes strongly unpleasant, your zinc levels are normal.

Good dietary sources for pregnant women include:

- red meat;
- seafood;
- brewer's yeast;
- wholegrain cereals;
- pulses;
- eggs;
- cheese.

EXERCISE

Exercise is an important part of staying fit and healthy during pregnancy, and in preparing you for childbirth. It also helps to boost circulation so more blood and nutrients pass through your placenta to reach your growing baby. It is important not to overexercise, however, as this will divert blood away from your baby to your muscles (to supply oxygen and energy) and to your skin (to cool you down). Aim to reduce your level of activity by around a third to 70 per cent of your level before you became pregnant.

As a general rule:

- try to exercise at least three times a week for at least 15 minutes;
- aim for gentle exercises such as walking, swimming or using an exercise bike;
- don't let your pulse rise above 120 beats per minute;
- don't let your body temperature rise above 37.8 °C (100°F);
- don't let yourself become dehydrated;
- avoid prolonged periods of aerobic exercise;
- stop if you become uncomfortable, short of breath or feel faint or tired;
- if you develop any complications of pregnancy (e.g. vaginal bleeding, contractions, or abdominal or chest pain) always seek medical advice about whether or not you can exercise.

From the fourth month of pregnancy onwards, avoid high impact sports such as jogging, sprinting or advanced aerobics, and activities where there is a risk of falling such as skiing or horse riding.

From five months of pregnancy onwards, your abdominal muscles will be stretched and you should avoid stomach exercises as these will place further strain on them. You should also avoid exercising flat on your back from the fifth month onwards as this can affect your circulation and cause dizziness.

Once your reach the sixth month of pregnancy, slowly start decreasing your level of exercise as you will be growing larger, and your balance will change. Towards the end of pregnancy, your ligaments will also start to soften and stretch owing to the effects of a hormone designed to help the birth canal widen during delivery. You can still do gentle non-weight-bearing exercise such as swimming, however, and can also practise yoga.

CHAPTER 3

Relaxation During Pregnancy

During pregnancy, mothers produce their own natural tranquilliser—a hormone known as pregnanolone—to help keep them relaxed and stress free. When you stop work and sit or lie down and relax, the muscles of your abdominal wall and womb relax too. Relaxation helps to optimise the flow of blood and nutrients to the womb and counteracts the potentially harmful effects of stress. Babies of mothers who take part in prenatal relaxation classes, such as yoga, have few obstetric complications and have a lower risk of having a low birth weight baby than do mothers who fail to relax regularly throughout pregnancy. Babies born to relaxed mothers are also less likely to suffer from anxiety, depression or hyperactivity in later life. It is therefore important to sit down for increasing periods of time as your pregnancy progresses. From around 30 weeks of pregnancy, it is also important to lie down for at least an hour mid-morning and mid-afternoon. Lying down relaxes the uterine muscles as well as boosting circulation through the placenta.

Try to stop working by around the 30th week of your pregnancy if you can. After this time, increased rest is vitally important for the health of both you and your growing baby. Prolonged standing and doing physical work for more than eight hours during the last three months of pregnancy can have the same damaging effect on your baby's development as heavy smoking, with babies weighing around 100 g less than those of women working 20 hours a week or less.

Keith Wright, acupuncturist and member of the International College of Oriental Medicine, especially advises women to rest when there is a full moon towards the end of pregnancy. He and local midwives have noticed that there is a greater tendency for premature breaking of waters at these times. According to one midwife 'The ward is full of broken waters when there is a full moon and low pressure weather. If the moon can pull on the tides, I'm damn sure it can break a few membranes!'

RELAXATION EXERCISES

The following quick exercise will help you to relax whenever you feel the need:

- Sit back comfortably in your chair.
- Raise both shoulders and circle them several times to stretch your shoulder muscles.
- Then let your shoulders drop and concentrate on relaxing any tension.
- Expand your chest and fill your lungs as far as possible.
- Breathe in and out deeply and slowly, concentrating on the rise and fall of your abdomen, not your chest.
- Repeat five times without holding your breath.
- Continue to breathe regularly, getting your rhythm right by slowly counting from one to three on breathing in and from one to four when breathing out.

The following longer exercise is excellent for helping you achieve total body relaxation. It is useful when you want to relax at the end of a highly stressful day, when you can't sleep and when you are preparing for meditation or visualisation. During the second half of pregnancy, when it becomes difficult to lie on your back, you can do this exercise in any semi-sitting, semi-reclining position that feels comfortable. It involves working many of the major muscle groups in your body, starting with the lower limbs. As you work the muscles learn to recognise the difference in feeling between tension and relaxation. Hold each constriction briefly and repeat each action twice with a short break in between.

- Find a warm, quiet place and lie down. Pull the curtains to dim the light.
- Loosen your clothing and relax on your back with head supported, arms and legs straight and slightly away from your body.
- Breathe in and out deeply for three breaths and imagine you are ridding your body of stress, then continue to breathe normally and close your eyes.
- Keeping your legs still, pull the upper part of your feet so your toes point as far forward as they can. Hold the tension, then release and feel the reduction in tension.
- Point your toes firmly away from your body and feel the tension in your calf muscles, hold, and then relax.
- Next draw your legs tightly towards you or raise them into the air, and hold, then drop them back to a relaxed position.
- Tense your buttocks by squeezing them hard together, hold, and then relax.
- Check your lower body is relaxed; it should feel heavy, warm and without tension.
- Now move your shoulders backwards to expand your chest, hold, and then release.
- Tense your shoulders by raising your arms and pulling on your shoulders, hold, and then relax.
- Now work on your hands and lower arms by making a tight fist, hold, then relax and let your fingers loosen. As you clench your fists for the second time raise your arms slightly off the ground and notice the tension in your forearms, hold, and then release.

- Move to the upper arms by bringing your hands towards your body, close to your chest, hold, and relax them down palms upwards.
- Relax your neck and throat by gently moving your head from side to side and then pulling your chin down to your chest, hold, and then release.
- Next clench your jaw by clamping your teeth together, hold, and then let go so that your mouth is slightly open.
- Now work on your facial muscles. Press your lips together, hold, and then release. Push your tongue hard to the roof of your mouth, hold, and then let it drop to the floor of your mouth.
- Without opening your eyes move them to the four quarters of a circle, and then let your eyelids relax.
- Finally relax your forehead and scalp. Frown hard and pull your forehead down, hold, and let go so that your face droops.

Your whole body should now feel heavy and relaxed. Breathe calmly and slowly and feel all the tension drain away. Imagine you are lying on a warm beach with a gentle breeze playing over your body. Relax for at least twenty minutes, occasionally checking your body for tension. In your own time, bring the session to a close.

VISUALISATION

Visualisation is a complementary technique that is similar to meditation but is easier to perform. Rather than trying to empty your mind of thought, you allow your mind to take you on an imagined journey to a quiet place where your desired outcome (e.g. a pain-free labour) can be fully visualised. It uses the power of suggestion and positive thought to help your desired, imagined goal turn into reality. Visualisation also helps to deepen relaxation, to overcome stress and to balance your emotions.

There are two types of visualisation: guided visualisation, in which a therapist or a relaxation tape leads your thoughts by instructing you on how to relax, and unguided visualisation, in which your own wandering thoughts guide your inner journey.

A visualisation exercise

Sit down comfortably in a quiet room with the curtains drawn. Imagine looking through a window into a lush, tranquil garden with foliage in restful shades of green, yellow, blue and white. Aromatic tropical flowers scent the air with vanilla, jasmine and rose as golden sunlight filters down, dappling you in restful cool shade, while the leaves of exotic palms and giant ferns steam gently in the heat. Use your senses to explore the colours, sounds and smells of this secret world as you drift deeper and deeper into a relaxed, meditative state.

You can use visualisation to help you prepare for labour by imagining contractions as a band around your abdomen that you effortlessly loosen and allow to fall away. When it is time to bring your inner journey to an end, imagine yourself walking in through your front door and closing it behind you, before opening your eyes, stretching your limbs and rejoining the present.

Using a mandala

A mandala is a popular Eastern device for guiding visualisation or meditation and helping you achieve a relaxed state. The name derives from a Sanskrit word meaning 'circle'. Each mandala is an intricate diagram composed of concentric circles, surrounded by an outer enclosure to represent the universe. Other symbols, geometric shapes and images of gods are usually included. Eastern mandalas are basically of two types, representing different aspects of the universe. When using a *garbha-dhatu* mandala, the eye moves across the images from the one to the many; while the *vajra-dhatu* mandala guides the eye from the many into the one. Concentrating on the images on a mandala can help you achieve a guided visualisation or a meditative state. If you prefer, you can use a favourite, intricate picture in a similar way.

Affirmations and visualisation

One of the most successful visualisation techniques is designed to be carried out just before you go to bed. This allows your subconscious mind to dwell on what you desire during sleep and improves the chance of a successful outcome.

1 Choose an appropriate positive affirmation such as: 'I am looking forward to a fulfilling and pain-free birth'.
2 Every night, when you go to bed, imagine your baby being born in a calm, relaxed, joyful and enjoyable, pain-free way.
3 Feel your love for the baby growing inside you as you welcome it into your heart and family.
4 Repeat your positive thought slowly and carefully to yourself.
5 Now touch the bed with the little finger of your left hand. Repeat the thought and touch the bed with the ring finger of your left hand while concentrating on the warm, loving glow you will feel when your baby is eventually born in an easy and pain-free labour.
6 Continue repeating your affirmation, while touching the bed with each finger (and thumb) of the left hand, and then the right. Then reverse the process, touching the bed starting with the little finger of the right hand.

By the time you have finished, you will have repeated the thought 20 times. Repeat this procedure every night for a week, staying awake throughout the entire process. The following week, repeat the process but let yourself fall asleep when you are ready. The statement should now have become part of your normal thinking patterns and you will have mentally prepared yourself for a fulfilling and pain-free labour.

Activating your *tan tien*
In the Chinese practice of qigong (see p. 142), a popular visualisation and relaxation exercise is the activation of the *tan tien* (*dan tian*); this is an area located about 5 cm (2 in) or three to four finger-breadths below the navel, and is considered to be the seat of the 'constitutional essence', termed *jing*. One aspect of *jing* nourishes a developing baby in the womb and is vital for growth and development. Your own *jing* can be strengthened by activating the *tan tien* through qigong— exercises utilising controlled breathing, combined with adjustment of body posture and focused awareness/visualisation. When the *tan tien* is activated, you may feel vibration and warmth in the area below the umbilicus. A useful Chinese technique to activate the *tan tien* is known as the 'inner smile':

- Sit comfortably with your back straight and your arms relaxed at your sides.
- Imagine something that makes you smile—perhaps the baby growing inside you.
- Allow yourself to smile internally so it is felt only by you and your baby—the smile does not have to be visible to anyone else.
- Let the smile shine out of your eyes and travel inwards to spread all over your body and into your baby, before concentrating just below your navel in the *tan tien*—the seat of your constitutional essence, or *jing*.
- As the smile radiates within, notice how relaxed and calm you feel.
- Once you feel relaxed yet energised, you can continue what you were previously doing, enriched by feelings of warmth, harmony and inner strength.

Visualisation during pregnancy

Keith Wright, lecturer at the International College of Oriental Medicine, describes below his use of visualisation during pregnancy:

I have been experimenting with visualisations to help women sort out some of their pregnancy problems. There are usually women in a panic who come needing to induce their labour, or to turn their breech babies before an imminent hospital deadline. By relaxing the mother with a gentle breathing technique, I have found that she will then be able to place her awareness down into her abdomen to feel the state of her uterus and the position and occupation of her baby at that time. By placing my hand on her tummy, I can feel and assist her in seeing what is going on. If the baby feels disinterested or unaware, or perhaps even distressed by the mother's predicament, it can be contacted via the heart–uterus connection (see Opening up your heart–uterus connection, below) and be properly informed.

Sometimes the baby's head is poorly positioned on the cervix. The mother will be able to know and often can tell in what way the head needs to move for improved contact. Again, I have had a lot of success in helping the mother to encourage the baby to move its head over and increase the pressure. Once the baby has been aligned, I usually ask the mother to use her breathing technique to draw energy through the walls of the uterus, from the cervix upwards to the apex, imitating the path of a contraction wave, and then to breathe out, down through the baby and cervix into the earth. In this way, we can map out with each full breath the path of the contractions and of the baby's route to the outside world, in preparation for the onset of labour. Finally, the baby can be encouraged to bear down on to the cervix to initiate contractions. The results have been very individual but always positive. Some women have gone directly into labour within a day. Others have discovered that they have big emotional blocks about their new baby, which they can then consider remedying. Whether or not the outcome is the actual onset of labour depends on the fundamental issue of how wholehearted is the mother's commitment to the birth and to the baby. This is the message that needs to be understood and absorbed into obstetric care. It demands that we ask, how can we ensure that each mother is as wholeheartedly content as possible, during her pregnancy and labour? We must ask this, not for the mother's sake alone. Remember, the well-being of her new baby, and its determination to initiate the various birth stimuli, depends upon her state of mind and body.

Opening up your heart–uterus connection

One of the most important things for an expectant mother to do is to open up her heart–uterus connection.

When a woman becomes pregnant, a channel or line of communication opens up between her 'heart' and that of her baby. The 'heart' in Chinese terms is the abode of the spirit, and is more akin to the heart centre (chakra) where we feel love and process the truth about life, as we perceive it, than to the organ that pumps blood round our bodies. The mother therefore has a way of knowing what her baby is doing and the baby understands the truth of what is in its mother's heart. For the baby, its mother is its lifeline and the only support it has are the intuited feelings from its mother via the line of communication. If the baby perceives that for some reason mum isn't wholeheartedly concentrated in giving birth, the baby may oblige her by not doing anything to initiate it. I believe that the act of inverting and engaging the head in the pelvis is a symbolic act of acceptance that the birth process should start, as much as the necessity of biology. If the baby feels that mum isn't ready to start the birth process, it will be less willing to engage its head. This is very often the cause of a breech baby or a pregnancy that goes well beyond its due

46

date. I have used this concept time and again with success in my clinics and the implications, for the whole of obstetric care, are immense. In some cases, breech babies have turned spontaneously following just a phone call in which it was explained to the mother the significance to her baby of her putting too much of her attention on other issues and not preparing emotionally for the birth.

Why should the baby take so much notice of its mother's wishes? For the baby, birth is the time when it has to leave behind everything it knows, all its resources of comfort, nourishment and perhaps most of all its mother's love. In fact, the Chinese say birth is 'leaving home'. For the baby, its birth-day is the day when it makes a huge leap of faith and undergoes a rite of passage to the 'other side' where it has little idea of what awaits it. Very largely, it is the strength of its mother's heart that gives the baby the encouragement to initiate the birth process.

It is vital that, for a good birth, the mother needs to be strong-hearted about the prospect. This implies too that she should have enough physical vitality, know her own mind about her birthing options, have the support and environment that she feels happy with for the birth, and not have any great worries or stresses that take her attention away from the consuming event that is soon to happen.

The concept of a mother's urge to nest is also vital to the success of her delivery. Animals seek a safe corner to hide up in, where they feel secure from the dangers of the world to have their babies. We, too, need a safe nest. In our society the emphasis is more often on mental safety; our nest is a feeling of security—a safe, emotional, mental space that a woman knows she can create when delivering her baby. This does not come without weeks of preparation and decision-making, and involves:

● resolving, where possible, any external issues that draw on her time and attention to the detriment of the baby;

- communication with and building a loving bond with the baby; this two-way knowing creates an unshakeable confidence between the birthing pair, and holds much sway in the conduct of the baby during the birth process.

As a result, a woman can face her forthcoming labour with strength, which she imparts to the baby. Mothers who:

- work until close to their due date;
- are in any way unsettled in the months and days approaching birth;
- are cajoled into accepting routine delivery procedures, against their wishes, without there being a clear medical necessity;

are likely candidates for disruption to their late pregnancies.

We must understand that it is the baby's birth, and that the mother is there only to labour for it. The baby is not a passive bundle with no mind or will of its own until it is born. It needs to be consulted and taken on board, so as to create a team with the mother, otherwise difficulties will arise and so often end up in the hands of the obstetrician on duty. Every time I do this sort of work with pregnant women, I am amazed at their sensitivity and awareness. It seems incredible to me that so many can feel the mood of their baby and its position in the uterus. Many relax into the meditation and, although I am their guide, they find their power and use it to full effect.

For the sake of the new babies, whose first moments are entrusted to our care, mothers *must* be treated with the greatest care and compassion. They *must* feel secure and confident in the nests of their hearts.

AUTOGENIC TRAINING AND PREGNANCY

Autogenic training (AT) is a complementary relaxation therapy that is becoming more popular, and can be used successfully during pregnancy. Nasim Kanji, Senior Lecturer, Faculty of

Health Studies, Buckinghamshire Chilterns University College, and a therapist in autogenic training and Honorary Secretary of the British Autogenic Society, explains how autogenic training can be helpful during pregnancy:

What autogenic training is

Autogenic training is a relaxation technique carried out by an individual on himself or herself, which involves the use of passive concentration and certain combinations of mental and physical stimuli. AT is defined medically as a form of psychotherapy.

Autogenic training was introduced in 1932 by Johannes Schultz and subsequently developed further by Wolfgang Luthe. Essentially it consists of a series of simple mental exercises designed to turn off the stress mechanisms in the body, and to turn on the restorative rhythms associated with profound mental and physical relaxation.

Autogenic training is self-induced, as its name implies, generated by a person from within, who is able to achieve a steadily developing enhancement of energy and tranquillity. Once learned, and this is a simple process, it may be practised for a lifetime. Carried out regularly and properly, AT can achieve results comparable to those attained by Eastern meditators who have been working at their practices for a long time. From the Western point of view, AT has the great appeal of being without cultural, religious or cosmological overtones or the requirement of special clothing, unusual postures or rituals.

Basic achievements of AT are the containment of stress and the alleviation of stress-related conditions such as sleep disorders, panic attacks, high blood pressure, asthma, phobias, muscular pain and tension, migraine, fatigue, menstrual disorders, aggression and unresolved grief. But AT offers more than this. By supporting the existing self-healing and self-regulating physiological functions of various body systems (homeostasis), AT facilitates and boosts the inherent self-healing properties of these systems. Further, AT enables an individual to become aware of physical, mental and spiritual manifestations that are varied and welcome, and also to become aware of recurrent negative patterns that diminish the quality of life. AT shows even the most dispirited person that there *are* alternatives and there

49

are choices, and, by operating on the principle 'what the mind causes, the mind can cure', it opens the door to a new and successful way of thinking and living.

Pregnancy—where autogenic training can help

Autogenic training offers a number of therapeutic advantages that are valuable in the pre- and postnatal periods and during labour. Often patients feel reassured simply because they have a technique at their disposal that is able to provide almost instant calmness and relaxation. However, it has been recognised that regular practice of the autogenic standard exercises, if started during the early phases of pregnancy, will also help women to cope with many of the standard disorders of pregnancy, and complaints such as nausea, vomiting, constipation, insomnia, shortness of breath, tenseness and irritability become less disturbing, and subside more quickly, under the influences of the standard exercises. Fear and anxiety of actual birth may also be relieved. In addition to helping with a patient's prenatal state, passive concentration on the first four standard AT formulae has been found to be beneficial in different stages of labour. Other favourable physiological changes take place with respect to blood pressure, heart rate, reduction of muscular tension and pain perception. The allaying of fatigue and exhaustion have also been noted.

For obvious reasons, and particularly because of the prophylactic and therapeutic value of autogenic training during the prenatal period, it is recommended that the patient begin with the standard AT exercises as early as possible after pregnancy is verified, or even during the pre-conceptual preparation period.

The autogenic training method

The basic autogenic training exercises are simple. There are three optional postures, namely:

- sitting slumped rag-doll style on a stool;
- lounging in an easy chair;
- lying prostrate, arms by the side.

Having ensured there will be no disturbances, the person takes up one of these postures. The eyes are closed and attention is focused on each arm in turn, right-handed people commencing with the suggestion: 'My right arm is heavy'. The principal theme of this first exercise is muscular relaxation.

Subsequent concentration is on warmth, which is keyed by the instruction: 'My right arm is warm', which instigates a developing situation whereby warmth is felt progressively in the other limbs until all the extremities become heavy and warm.

After having learned how to induce a feeling of heaviness and warmth, the trainee is taught passive concentration on cardiac activity through use of the formula: 'My heartbeat is calm and regular'. Then follows passive concentration on the respiratory mechanism with the formula: 'It breathes me', after which the person focuses on warmth in the abdominal region with: 'My solar plexus is warm'. The final standard exercise concerns the cranial region, which should be cooler than the rest of the body, and here the formula is: 'My forehead is cool'. The time needed to establish these exercises with a trainee varies between eight and ten weeks.

The effectiveness of passive concentration on a given formula is seen to depend on two other factors: the first is mental contact with the part of the body indicated by the formula, for example the right arm; the second is representation of the autogenic formula in the mind. At the outset, passive concentration on a formula should not last more than thirty to sixty seconds, and should lead only to superficial relaxation. The time span is gradually increased, with an increasing depth of relaxation, to ten to fifteen minutes. Apprehension must be avoided, as must any goal-directed effort.

The state of passive concentration is terminated by the application of a three-step procedure: the arms are flexed energetically; the trainee breathes deeply; the eyes are opened.

Learning autogenic training

Although autogenic training is a simple, straightforward technique, the British Autogenic Society recommend that it is learned under full supervision of Autogenic Training Therapists who have undergone a specialised training course. A list of qualified therapists may be obtained from the British Autogenic Society (see Useful Addresses, p. 226).

FLOATATION THERAPY

Floatation therapy is a wonderful alternative technique to help you achieve deep relaxation. It involves lying in a lightproof, sound-insulated tank containing a shallow (ten inch deep) pool of warm water in which 700 lb of Epsom salts (magnesium sulphate) are dissolved. This forms a supersaturated solution of saline, which is kept at a constant skin temperature of 93.5 °F (34.5 °C). The floater is suspended on this bed of minerals, which, as it is more buoyant than the Dead Sea, neutralises many of the effects of gravity. This is important in helping you achieve relaxation as it is estimated that 90 per cent of all brain activity is concerned with the effects of gravitational pull on the body (e.g. correcting posture, maintaining balance, etc.). The tank screens out light and sound so your brain is cut off from virtually all external stimulation. This induces a profoundly relaxed state in which you generate the special brainwaves—theta waves—associated with meditation, creative thought and feelings of serenity. Studies show that you also continue to produce large amounts of theta waves for up to three weeks after a float.

Floatation therapy is beneficial throughout pregnancy, and specially during the last few months when it is the only time in which you can comfortably lie on your back! Many of the beneficial effects of floatation therapy are due to a significant fall in blood levels of stress hormones—a fall that is maintained for up to five days after treatment has stopped. Floatation has been shown to lower high blood pressure even after a single float lasting 45 minutes. This effect continues gradually across repeated sessions, and the lower blood pressure is maintained after floatation therapy stops. Control studies using subjects reclining in dimly lit, quiet rooms do not show the same effects, so it is not merely the process of relaxation inducing the measured changes. Floatation therapy also increases secretion of endorphins, which are opiates, or morphine-like substances, that are the brain's natural painkillers. This reduces chronic pain, produces feelings of euphoria and also improves the quality of sleep. Floatation therapy has, in addition, been found to reduce secretion of antidiuretic hormone so that excess retained fluid is lost by the production of larger quantities of urine shortly after a float.

Floatation therapy has been described as a return to the womb as you are floating in a warm salt solution in an enclosed, dark yet safe place from which you will eventually have to emerge into the world. The increased secretion of endorphins also mimics that which occurs in pregnancy when the levels are up to eight times higher than normal. The baby is exposed during pregnancy to these higher levels which have a soothing stress-reducing effect. This soothing effect may be reproduced as a 'womb-memory' that helps to sooth adults during floatation, too.

Floatation can help to reduce several pregnancy-associated problems such as headache, high blood pressure, back pain and fatigue. It is also helpful for those who have given up smoking and still experience some nicotine cravings.

During floatation, you can also learn to focus in on your own body—a technique known as biofeedback. Some people learn to regulate body functions that are not usually under voluntary control such as speeding or slowing the heart rate at will and reducing a raised blood pressure. During pregnancy, focusing inwards will also help you to bond and communicate with your baby.

Most people prefer to float naked, but you can wear a bathing costume if you wish. You will be given earplugs to wear to protect your ears from the very salty solution, and should also apply Vaseline to cuts as the solution will sting if it comes into contact with open skin wounds. Take great care not to drip any of the saline into your eyes as this will sting greatly. It is important to have professional supervision during floating when you are pregnant or if you are susceptible to claustrophobia. Floatation is not usually advised for those with a history of psychosis or epilepsy.

For best results, try a course of five weekly floats. You can obtain a similar deep relaxation in your own bathroom using mineral salts from the Dead Sea (available from larger health food stores and pharmacies). After soaking for 20 minutes, lie down in a warm, darkened, quiet room to fall asleep.

YOGA

Yoga is an oriental therapy that uses postural exercises, breathing techniques, meditation and relaxation to improve joint suppleness and overall health, and to relieve stress. During pregnancy, yoga helps to maintain flexibility and to relieve back pain. By encouraging rest and relaxation it also boosts blood flow through the placenta so more oxygen and nutrients can reach the baby. Research has shown that women who took part in prenatal relaxation classes, such as yoga, had fewer problems during pregnancy and have a lower risk of a low birth weight baby than those who do not relax regularly throughout pregnancy.

Yoga is an important part of the active birth movement, which was founded in the late 1970s by Janet Balaskas. She describes her philosophy below:

The active birth movement
The active birth movement encourages women to use upright positions and remain mobile during labour instead of lying or semi-reclining in bed. The approach is practical with the emphasis on preparation of both body and mind, as well as on-going emotional support throughout pregnancy.

Pregnant women are encouraged to join active birth classes as early as possible in pregnancy, although it is never too late to join. You will be invited to attend a weekly class of easy and relaxing 'gravitational' yoga, which is non-strenuous, can be done without previous experience and is ideally suited for pregnancy. These yoga-based exercises help to relieve tightness and tension in the body, improve flexibility, and encourage good breathing and circulation. They also relieve many of the common complaints of pregnancy, such as back ache or cramps, and are emotionally supportive and deeply relaxing. Besides helping to make pregnancy more healthy and enjoyable, these classes offer effective practical preparation for labour and birth. You will learn to be comfortable in upright positions and to manage pain in labour with breathing and relaxation. The classes may also offer informative courses or workshops that aim to increase the potential for a natural birth and breast feeding, whilst introducing expectant parents to a wide range of possibilities and options. They have an open-minded approach, covering the same ground as traditional antenatal classes, with an additional emphasis on upright labour and birth positions, relaxation, breathing and the use of warm water during labour and possibly also for birth.

After your baby is born, Active Birth teachers offer ongoing support in the form of postnatal yoga classes, in which you can meet up with mums from your pregnancy class. Many of them include baby massage, which may help to relieve colic and fretfulness and encourage your baby to sleep better. The Active Birth Centre also offers a water birth pool hire service.

For further information, read *Active Birth* by Janet Balaskas (Thorsons) or contact the Active Birth Centre (see Useful Addresses, p. 221).

The Yoga for Health Foundation also encourages the use of yoga during pregnancy and describes its benefits below:

Yoga during pregnancy

Yoga, which includes breathing practices, postures, relaxation and meditation, brings about a feeling of contentment and well-being in the practitioner. Pregnancy is a time of great change—physically, mentally and emotionally. Yoga can bring benefits on all these levels, benefiting both the mother and the child.

Some of the problems that may occur during pregnancy can be avoided. For example, back ache is eased, and the muscles of the back are strengthened. Standing poses tone up leg muscles, and help to prevent varicose veins. Postures known as the 'asanas' regulate the functioning of the glands and internal organs, improving the circulation of blood and lymph, and the distribution of oxygen to the tissues. The body is strengthened and prepared for the hard work of labour, and the flexibility achieved helps the mother to find the best position for the birth—for example, squatting or kneeling. During the birth, being able to relax during the contractions, and to control and use the breath, is of great help. Meditation brings calmness and inner peace, and helps the mother to have confidence in her new role. The general increase in awareness generated by the practice of yoga enhances the loving relationship between mother and unborn child.

If the mother has not practised yoga before, it is best not to start until after the third month of pregnancy, as in the early stages the risk of miscarriage is greater. It is best to start with a teacher who is used to teaching pregnant women. (At Ickwell Bury we run a course for yoga teachers who wish to learn more about yoga in pregnancy. This is taught by a midwife who is also a yoga teacher.)

If the mother is already practising, she will be able to carry on with her usual routine. When working on the asanas, avoid any pressure on the abdomen, or practices that increase pressure in the abdominal cavity.

The changes in hormone levels in pregnancy cause a loosening of the ligaments, particularly in the pelvis. Therefore in asanas the student must be encouraged to listen to the body, paying great attention to how she feels in each posture, and not to overstretch, as this could result in the joints becoming unstable later.

Baddha Konasana is probably the most important asana to practise during pregnancy, as it involves stretching and opening the pelvic floor. Pelvic congestion is relieved, and it may help to prevent gynae-cological problems in later life. Squatting is also useful.

A practical session
1   Lie on the back with the legs up the wall. (This helps to tone the leg muscles and prevent varicose veins.)
2   Take the legs wide apart up the wall; hold for 30 breaths.

3 Then bend the knees, bringing the soles of the feet together, with the outside edges of the feet against the wall (*Baddha Konasana*—Cobbler pose). Hold for 15 breaths.

4 Bring the knees to the chest, roll on to one side and over into the 'pose of the child', with the knees apart. Make fists with the hands, and support the head on the fists. Hold for 10 breaths.

5 Go on to the hands and knees.

6 Sit with the back to the wall, in *Baddha Konasana*. Breathe down to the baby.

7 Move on to the hands and knees for the 'cat' movement. (Lift the tailbone, hollow the back, lift the head on inhalation, and tuck under the tail and head on exhalation.) Then circle the pelvis with the breath.

8 Standing poses. Choose from:
   Tadasana (Mountain pose);
   Virabhadrasana 1 (Warrior pose);
   Virabhadrasana 2;
   Parsvakonasana—Extended lateral angle pose (on to thigh);
   Uttanasana—standing forward bend pose (hands on to ledge);
   Foot on ledge, with a hamstring stretch.

9 Squatting, holding on to a partner or heavy furniture for support.

10 Gentle twist:
   first stage of *Marichyasana* 1 (Sitting twist pose)
   Bharadvajasana 1 (Sitting twist pose).
   Twist, sitting on a chair.

11 Deep breathing, sitting cross legged.

12 Relaxation. (Avoid lying on the back, as the weight of the uterus presses on the vena cava, causing the blood pressure to drop. A modified recovery position, with cushions for support where necessary, can be used.)

Several different forms of yoga are available. According to Louis Pivcevic of the Yoga Biomedical Trust:

The yoga pioneered by Dr Françoise Freedman adapts traditional asanas and breathing to facilitate a fit, relaxed pregnancy and a birth without undue strain, resistance or fear.

Yogic breathing uniquely connects the action of the voluntary and involuntary muscles in the abdomen, giving the woman more control over all her movements. By expanding breathing and stretching capacity, women gain greater confidence and control through familiarity with the muscles used in birth. This is especially important for first-time mothers.

Other benefits include improved posture, both ante- and postnatal. There is a more rapid recovery of good muscle tone after the birth. As a new mother you will enjoy your baby more because you will feel fit and rested. You can also expect better gynaecological health in later life (prevention of prolapse and incontinence) because you have learnt how to look after your body during pregnancy. Lastly, by practising deep abdominal breathing you are providing the unborn baby with a richer supply of blood and stimulating its body at the same time. The deep relaxation and meditation practised at the end of each session helps deepen the emotional bonds between mother and baby, as well as nurturing the mother's sense of self and identity.

The Yoga Therapy Centre also offers combined postnatal and baby yoga classes. These use the weight of the baby to tone the mother's body and during these classes find their bodies become stronger, fitter and more supple than before pregnancy. Baby massage is also integrated into the postnatal programme.

The Yoga Therapy Centre also offers unique ante- and post-natal aquayoga classes, where yoga stretches and breathing are greatly enhanced by practising in the warm water of a swimming pool.

CHAPTER 4

Exploring Complementary Therapies

Complementary therapies are an increasingly popular adjunct or even alternative to conventional medicine. Their holistic approach in treating mind, body and spirit comes from the realisation that physical health stems from emotional balance. By encouraging a more positive frame of mind, complementary techniques offer a gentler and safer form of healing.

The following complementary therapies can help many women during pregnancy, but, just as with orthodox medicine, not every treatment will suit every individual. Some therapies can be used for self-help, whilst for others you will need to consult a therapist. This is especially important to ensure that only herbs and essential oils known to be safe are taken during pregnancy.

When choosing an alternative practitioner, bear in mind that standards of training and experience vary widely. Where possible:

- Select a therapist on the basis of personal recommendation from a satisfied client whom you know and whose opinion you trust.
- Check what qualifications the therapist has, and check the therapist's standing with the relevant umbrella organisation for that therapy. The organisation will be able to tell you what training their members have undertaken, inform you

of their code of ethics and refer you to qualified practitioners in your area.
- Find out how long your course of treatment will last and how much it is likely to cost.
- Ask how much experience the therapist has had in treating women during pregnancy and what the success rate is for any particular pregnancy-associated problem.
- Ask about the extent of experience in treating pregnancy-associated conditions in general.

ACUPUNCTURE

Acupuncture is an ancient therapy that has been practised in the Orient for four to five thousand years. It is based on the belief that life energy (*ch'i* or *qi*—pronounced 'chee') flows through your body along different channels called 'meridians'. Classic acupuncture is based on the belief that the flow of energy depends on the balance of two opposing forces: the *yin* and the *yang*—a balance which is easily disrupted through factors such as stress, emotions, poor diet and spiritual neglect. When this 'energy flow' becomes blocked, symptoms of illness are triggered. There are 12 main meridians—six of which have a *yang* polarity and are related to hollow organs (e.g. womb), and six are *yin* relating mainly to solid organs (e.g. liver). Eight further meridians control the other 12. Along each meridian a number of acupoints have been identified where *ch'i* energy is concentrated and can enter or leave the body. Three hundred and sixty-five classic acupoints were traditionally sited on the meridians but many more have now been discovered—around 2000 acupoints are illustrated on modern charts. Researchers can now identify acupoints with a simple, hand held machine that measures electrical potentials across the skin. Acupoints have been found to have a lower electrical resistance than surrounding areas and can be pinpointed with great accuracy to place acupuncture onto a more scientific footing.

Keith Wright, who is a member of the British Acupuncture Council and a traditional acupuncture practitioner who specialises in pregnancy, explains:

The physical body is hung upon an energy framework, part of which is the system of acu-meridians. By balancing the energy in the system, you alter the function of the physical body, since the physical depends upon the energetic for its life. In my experience, most problems encountered in pregnancy and childbirth are due to:

- poor vitality of the energy body leading to weakness or dysfunction in the physical;
- energy blockages in the meridians, which lead to imbalance in the energy flow and in the physical balance.

A therapist can stimulate, alter or unblock the flow of *ch'i* by inserting fine, disposable needles into specific acupuncture points, depending on your individual symptoms, the appearance of your tongue, and on the quality, rhythm and strength of 12 pulse positions on the radial artery—six in each wrist—which are recognised in Chinese medicine. These pulses help to identify areas where the flow of *ch'i* is blocked. The best known effect of *ch'i* manipulation is in pain relief (local anaesthesia) and research suggests that acupuncture stimulates release of the body's own natural painkillers.

According to Dr Richard Halvorsen, a GP and member of the British Medical Acupuncture Society:

The term acupuncture may refer to at least four different therapies, each with different principles:

1 Classical acupuncture based on the historical Chinese philosophical ideas of '*yin* and *yang*', 'five elements' and flow of *ch'i* (energy) along meridians.
2 Scientific acupuncture: a Westernised version of acupuncture in which treatment is given based on modern scientific understanding.
3 Acupuncture as a form of trigger point therapy.
4 Electroacupuncture, in which the needles are stimulated electrically.

Acupuncture used in pregnancy and childbirth may involve any or several of these approaches which can be combined to good effect. Experience and, to some extent, research demonstrate that acupuncture has plenty to offer both the women going through a normal pregnancy and also the woman who needs help with one or more problems surrounding pregnancy or childbirth.

Inserting a needle a few millimetres into the skin causes little if any discomfort. You may notice a slight pricking sensation, tingle or buzz as the needle is inserted or rotated. According to Dr Halvorsen, 'the fine metal needles are inserted into the skin to a depth of up to 4 cm. They will usually be left in place for up to 30 minutes (10–20 minutes would be typical) and sometimes stimulated with electricity or occasionally moxa—a strong-smelling Chinese herb (usually wild mugwort, *Artemisia vulgaris*).' Most patients notice an immediate benefit after just one or two treatments, while with others it may take up to four to six treatments.

What happens during a consultation?
Zita West is a midwife who also practises acupuncture and runs The Pregnancy Shop (see Useful Addresses, p. 220). She says:

Women are increasingly keen to know about the use of acupuncture for common ailments in pregnancy and for pain relief during labour. They are understandably reluctant to take drugs, and acupuncture is an obvious, drug-free choice with no side-effects. During a first appointment, which may take up to 90 minutes, a full case history is taken. Everything about the patient is relevant—age, lifestyle, emotional and physical traits—not just the problem she has come with. The functions of all her body systems are taken into account by thorough questions regarding appetite, digestion, bowel movements, circulation, sleep and energy levels. The tongue is examined and can provide important information; e.g. a yellow-coated tongue indicates internal heat, which needs to be cleared using the appropriate acupoints; a white-coated tongue suggests internal cold; redness may indicate heartburn. There are three pairs of pulse positions in each wrist, making 12 altogether. The relative differences between these indicate the energy balance of the body. The Chinese system of total or holistic diagnosis indicates which acupuncture points need to be accessed for an individually tailored treatment. Other factors are also taken into account; for example, morning sickness in which bile is brought up suggests liver disharmony, while sickness without bile suggests stomach and spleen disharmony, which requires treatment at different acupuncture points. Treating pregnant women requires great care as there are certain points that must be avoided because of the risk of miscarriage (e.g. Large Intestine 4 on the hand, and Spleen 6 on the inside of the leg.

Acupuncture remains one of the most widely used and effective complementary therapies during pregnancy. Dr Richard Halvorsen describes the main uses of medical acupuncture during pregnancy as follows.

Acupuncture during pregnancy and childbirth

Nausea of pregnancy

The nausea of pregnancy (early morning sickness) is, without doubt, helped greatly by acupuncture. It has been used for 4000 years for this purpose, and numerous scientific trials have proven that acupuncture really is effective in relieving this distressing, but all too common, 'side-effect' of pregnancy. The classic site for inserting the needles is Pericardium 6 (Neiguan or PC6) in the forearm (see p. 71), but other points may also be used.

Back ache and sciatica

These common pregnancy-related conditions are treated successfully by acupuncture. Often local 'trigger points' in the back will be used alongside more traditional acupuncture points. This is another area where modern scientific research has confirmed acupuncture's effectiveness.

Carpal tunnel syndrome

This painful condition affecting the hand, wrist and sometimes the forearm is due to the build-up of fluid during pregnancy. Though there is little objective evidence, acupuncture does appear to help relieve this painful problem, which usually settles on its own after delivery.[1]

Headaches

Headaches can be troublesome during pregnancy. If so, this is another condition where acupuncture can give benefit.

Constipation

Pregnant women suffer from constipation much more often than non-pregnant women. Those fortunate people who have never been constipated do not realise the pain and distress that this trivial-

---

[1] Zita West has found carpal tunnel syndrome can improve with daily acupuncture treatments, but patients remain pain free for only a couple of hours after each visit.

sounding problem can cause. Whilst diet should not be ignored, acupuncture can also help. Points used often include those on the Stomach and Large Intestine meridians.

Haemorrhoids
One unfortunate consequence of constipation can be haemorrhoids (piles), which can cause either painless bleeding on defaecation or quite severe pain when attempting to defaecate. This is another area where there is a lack of research, but acupuncture can help here.[1]

Varicosities
These can occur either in the legs or in the vulva. Along with other approaches, acupuncture may help.[2]

Breech
Moxibustion to point Bladder 67, at the outer corner of the little toenail, has long been used by acupuncturists to turn the fetus from the breech position in the womb to the 'head-first' position. A study published in the *Journal of the American Medical Association* in November 1998 reported on some research on women between 33 and 35 weeks of pregnancy who had fetuses in the breech position (i.e. bottom first). The results show that burning a moxa roll (a cigar-shaped stick containing the herb mugwort) over the acupuncture point Bladder 67 of these women significantly increased the chance of the baby turning to the normal 'head-first position. This may work by causing an increase in the fetal movements. It is undoubtedly a remarkably safe, easy, cheap and effective treatment.

Induction of delivery
Acupuncture, sometimes using electricity, can be used to increase uterine contractions. Some midwives will use this for women who are 'post-term'.

[1] Zita West has found acupuncture is highly successful for treating haemorrhoids during and after pregnancy.
[2] Zita West has found an Acutens machine, which stimulates acupuncture points electrically, works well when used along the leg meridians.

Pain relief during labour

Trials have shown both acupuncture and electroacupuncture to be effective in relieving the pain of childbirth. Electroacupuncture is particularly helpful, but is not ideal in labour because of the need to be attached to wires and the unpredictable pain relief achieved.

Pain relief in caesarian section

Research suggests that some women obtain significant pain relief from acupuncture during delivery by caesarian section. In practice, it is likely to be difficult to use this technique in the hospital environment, particularly with regard to emergency caesarian deliveries.

Normal pregnancy

Many traditional Chinese acupuncturists will offer acupuncture as a method of balancing the energy of the body and providing a harmonious relationship between the mother and her baby. Acupuncture may assist normal uterine contractions, possibly by improving its blood supply. Not surprisingly, there is no evidence to support its effectiveness in this regard. If you do seek this sort of treatment then do follow the cautions given below.

Other conditions

Acupuncture may also be helpful in the following conditions: prevention of miscarriage (use with caution—there is, as yet, no evidence that acupuncture does more good than harm), female infertility (due to hormone disorders), oedema of pregnancy, sleep disturbance and heartburn (indigestion).

Safety

Some acupuncturists are reluctant to use any acupuncture (as opposed to acupressure) in the first trimester of pregnancy, but complications are extremely rare in well-qualified and experienced hands.

Cautions: Moxibustion is generally not recommended in pregnancy (as it is believed to increase the *ch'i* of the uterus, which could, theoretically, lead to a miscarriage)—with the notable exception of its proven benefit in turning breech babies.

Certain specific acupuncture points should not be strongly stimulated in the pregnant woman, particularly in the first trimester; pregnant women in China are rarely treated with acupuncture before 12 weeks.

The abdomen should only be needled, if at all, with extreme caution during pregnancy. It should not be needled below the umbilicus during the first six months of pregnancy.

Acupuncture treatment should always be obtained from an experienced acupuncturist, but this is particularly important for the pregnant woman. In an ideal world the obstetrician or midwife herself would administer the acupuncture. Failing that, find an experienced acupuncturist through the professional bodies listed in the Useful Addresses section, pp. 222–5.

Availability

There are three units in the UK where midwives practise acupuncture on the NHS. So if you live near to Plymouth, Warwick or Central London you may be lucky enough to receive acupuncture from your midwife. A nominal fee may be charged for the needles. Although the use of acupuncture in the NHS is on the increase, you will most likely have to pay for any treatment you receive. Charges are very variable, ranging from 'what you can afford' to £50 or more a treatment.

Remember that expensive treatment does not necessarily mean better treatment. The most important thing is to find a qualified and experienced practitioner and not to take any chances.

For information on how to find an acupuncturist, see Useful Addresses. Most acupuncture in pregnancy is carried out in private clinics by registered professional acupuncturists.

Keith Wright (see p. 61) says that an acupuncturist present during a birth, whether at home or in hospital, can act as an independent helper to assist the progress of delivery and with the after-birth care. He describes his use of acupuncture in pregnancy as follows:

Acupuncture can help to maintain vitality and a sense of well-being throughout pregnancy. Traditionally, two special acupuncture treatments are given at the end of the third and sixth months to stabilise the fetus and to reinforce the mother's energies for the next trimester. Even if no other treatments are sought, these two can help greatly.

As well as helping to alleviate sickness during pregnancy, acupuncture can calm an irritated uterus and stop inappropriate contractions, which may help to reduce the risk of miscarriage. It can also be used to raise the placenta where it develops too close to the cervix (placenta previa), to reduce high blood pressure and to alleviate many common problems during pregnancy, including fatigue, cramps, cravings, constipation, heartburn, fluid retention, insomnia, piles, shortness of breath, anaemia and diabetes.

High blood pressure

The general results of using acupuncture for treating high blood pressure in pregnancy are very good, especially when there is no history of hypertension before the pregnancy. High blood pressure in pregnancy is usually linked with chronic low energy levels. The added load of being pregnant throws the body into emergency mode by tightening the blood vessels or increasing adrenaline levels so the body can hold itself together. A patient with an overall 'deficient' energy picture will suffer from sporadic hypertension as weakness causes her body to react to stressful daily situations by relying on frequent adrenaline surges. These can be alleviated by building her energy levels so blood pressure surges become less frequent. Similarly, a blockage in the flow of energy in the meridians causes the body to react in an emergency fashion, creating hypertension. Typical stimuli are:

- emotional tension/anger → bodily tension → blockage of energy;
- physical discomfort of pregnancy → pain → tension → blockage of energy flow.

Acupuncture can increase energy levels and help to overcome these effects. The root cause is generally fairly superficial and easily relieved with acupuncture.

Preparing for labour

It is important to open up your heart–uterus connection during pregnancy (see p. 46) and to initiate the nesting instinct during the last six or eight weeks of pregnancy so your baby feels able to initiate the birthing process. Acupuncture can encourage the baby's head to engage and can be used to induce labour at nature's pace, as an alternative to a hospital induction.

During labour

First stage of labour
During the first stage of labour, during which the cervix becomes fully dilated, acupuncture helps to relax and soften the cervix to aid its dilation. It helps to calm and stabilise the mother and baby during labour, control pain, and can reinforce the mother's energy levels to speed the first stage of labour if this is slow.

Second stage of labour
During the second stage of labour, in which the baby passes through the birth canal, acupuncture can strengthen weak uterine contractions to increase their efficiency in expelling the baby and can effectively manage the time-scale of the whole labour, as well as alleviating palpitations, breathlessness, upper abdominal pain and haemorrhaging.

Third stage of labour
During the third stage of labour, in which the placenta (afterbirth) is expelled, acupuncture can be used to induce the placenta to release from the uterus, relieve postdelivery pains and stem haemorrhaging.

Postnatal problems
Acupuncture is also helpful after childbirth in relieving postnatal depression, insomnia, urinary and bowel problems, as well as helping the mother to re-establish her balance of health. Acupuncture is also used to treat a caesarean scar, once healed, to regulate the flow of breast milk and to alleviate mastitis.

Zita West (see p. 62) says:

> The main points I use during labour are on the ear. Auricular acupuncture is the insertion of small needles into the outer ear where the acupuncture points are concentrated. For pain relief, three needles are used with electrodes attached to an electrical device similar to a TENS machine. Treatment can also be given to speed contractions, and relieve back pain and pains after delivery. Body acupoints are also used to boost the mother's energy during labour and to help prevent a prolonged labour. For turning a breech baby heat is applied by burning sticks of moxa close to a point on the little toe, which can be effective from 32 weeks on ...
>
> Acupuncture is rapidly losing its esoteric overtones, which is completely appropriate for a practical system of medicine which is based on 4000 years of use and empirical observation. I am delighted to see it becoming more available on the NHS and hope that the use of acupuncture in midwifery will continue to spread throughout the UK.

ACUPRESSURE

Acupressure is an ancient oriental technique practised in China and Japan for over 3000 years. Acupressure is similar to acupuncture, but, instead of inserting needles at points along the meridians to balance the flow of *qi* energy, the acupoints are stimulated using firm thumb pressure or fingertip massage. Sometimes the therapist will also use palms, elbows, knees and feet to stimulate different parts of your body.

There are three main forms of acupressure massage: tui na, shiatsu and zero balancing.

While you can use acupressure on yourself to help relieve minor conditions when not pregnant, in general only a specialist should practise acupressure on someone who is pregnant as certain points should not be stimulated during pregnancy. One point you can stimulate yourself, however, is Pericardium 6 (PC6), found on the wrist (see below). Twenty-seven different studies have shown that this point is effective in treating sickness due to a variety of causes, including pregnancy. In one survey, nearly 80 per cent of women suffering from morning sickness found their symptoms improved dramatically when they wore special acupressure bands designed to stimulate the PC6 point. No side-effects were reported. Dr Richard Halvorsen comments as follows:

Acupressure for nausea
Pressing for five minutes over PC6 (situated in the middle of the inner forearm, approximately the breadth of two thumbs above the wrist crease), either every two to three hours or whenever sickness is felt, has been shown to be helpful. The same effect can be obtained by wearing commercially available wrist bands with a stud pressing on point PC6. These are available from chemists.

Keith Wright advises that, as pregnancy progresses, more acupoints become contraindicated. In particular, he warns that, according to the classics, PC6 should not be used to relieve nausea after the eighth week of pregnancy.

ALEXANDER TECHNIQUE

The Alexander technique is based on the belief that poor posture and faulty body movements contribute to disease. Gentle exercises and movements teach you how to stand and move correctly, without undue stress. As well as improving physical co-ordination, the technique has an holistic approach that also addresses mental and emotional function. By improving the quality of thinking, and attending to how tasks are performed, the method helps to reduce strain and conserve energy.

Pregnancy is a time when body posture and the centre of gravity change. The principles of Alexander technique can help you adjust to these changes; it is beneficial for a wide variety of pregnancy-associated conditions, but especially back and pelvic pain, high blood pressure, fatigue, digestive problems, stress, anxiety and low spirits. Alexander technique teachers also encourage pelvic floor exercises in preparation for childbirth, and recommend that women stay upright during labour so gravity can naturally assist the birthing process.

The technique teaches you how to consciously release tension so you can remain relaxed and experience reduced pain perception throughout the process of birth. To learn it, you will usually need a minimum course of 30 lessons, each lasting around 30–45 minutes.

AROMATHERAPY

Aromatherapy has been practised for at least 4000 years and was popular in Ancient India, Greece, Rome and Egypt. Aromatic essential oils are produced by special glands in the leaves, stems, bark, flowers, roots or seeds of certain plants. These oils contain many active ingredients in a highly concentrated and potent form that, because they are volatile, readily evaporate to release their powerful scent. The oils are collected in a variety of ways. Those extracted by simple pressing (e.g. bergamot, lemon, orange) are known as 'essences', those extracted by distillation are known as 'essential oils', while those obtained by enfleurage (pressing petals between glass sheets coated with animal fat) and solvent extraction are correctly known as 'absolutes'. The term 'essential oil' is commonly used to describe them all, however.

Every day when you are breathing and sniffing, over 10 000 different aromatic chemicals are wafted up towards receptors at the top of the nose. These aromas are detected by hair-like nerve endings that, unlike those involved in other senses, are directly connected to the brain, so messages from the nose are passed directly to the limbic system without being filtered by higher centres. Smells can therefore have a profound effect on emotions and behaviour as they can trigger primitive responses that have not been modified by intellectual input. The limbic system is also one of the most ancient parts of the brain and is directly linked to other centres involved in learning, memories, arousal, emotions and hormone secretion. As a result, the sense of smell can trigger powerful responses such as hunger, nostalgia, fear and mood changes, as well as playing an important role in the recognition and bonding interactions that occur between mother and baby.

Essential oils are highly concentrated and—with a few exceptions—should always be diluted with a carrier oil (e.g. avocado, calendula, grapeseed, jojoba, sunflower or wheatgerm oil) before being placed on the skin. Once in contact with the skin, some of the oils' constituents will be absorbed to have a medicinal effect in the body. Excess of some oils may be harmful—especially during pregnancy—so always choose oils carefully (preferably with the assistance of a qualified aromatherapist) and follow the instructions that come with the pack.

Where possible, use natural rather than synthetic essential oils. Natural oils generally have a fuller, sweeter aroma that provides a greater therapeutic benefit. Similarly, 100 per cent pure essential oils, whilst more expensive, are more desirable as they have not been mixed with alcohol or other additives.

Dilution
Essential oils should always be diluted in a carrier oil before massaging into the skin or adding to bath water. This dilution is important as oils that are too concentrated may have an adverse effect or cause skin irritation. When making your own essential oil blends add one drop of essential oil per 5 ml (one medicinal teaspoon) to make a 1 per cent solution. For larger quantities:

add a total of 10 drops essential oils to 100 ml carrier oil to produce a 0.5 per cent solution;
add a total of 20 drops essential oils to 100 ml carrier oil to produce a 1 per cent solution;
add a total of 40 drops essential oils to 100 ml carrier oil to produce a 2 per cent solution.

Aromatherapy uses a variety of techniques to obtain therapeutic benefit from essential oils. They may be inhaled, massaged into the skin, added to bath water, or heated in a variety of ways to perfume the atmosphere and produce a therapeutic atmosphere.

Methods of use

Massage oil
Add essential oils to carrier oil according to the dilution advised, and mix thoroughly before massaging into the skin. (See p. 134 on how to give a massage.)

Massage lotion/cream
Add essential oils to a neutral (non-scented) body lotion or cream according to the dilution advised, and mix thoroughly before massaging into the skin.

Bathing
Draw your bath so that it is comfortably warm (not too hot) but do not add the aromatherapy oils until the taps are turned off. Add a tablespoon (15 ml) of diluted essential oil and mix. Close the bathroom door to keep in the vapours and soak for 15–20 minutes, preferably in candlelight.

Showering
After cleansing your body with soap or gel, rinse well then dip a wet sponge in the diluted essential oil mix and use it to massage your whole body gently while under a warm jet spray.

Perfume
Dab diluted oil behind your ears, in your cleavage, under your breasts and on your wrists.

Pot pourri
Add a few drops of undiluted essential oils to a pot pourri mix to scent your bedroom. Refresh the scent regularly as it starts to fade.

Room spray
Fill a small sprayer with 100 ml water and add ten drops of your chosen undiluted essential oils. Shake the sprayer well before using it to perfume a room. This mix can also be placed in special porous holders that will sit over a radiator.

Candle diffuser
Add a few drops of your chosen undiluted essential oils to hot water in the top of the diffuser then light the candle underneath so the scented water starts to vaporise.

Ring burner
An aromatherapy ring burner is designed to sit over a light bulb so the oils it contains are gently diffused by the heat energy of the bulb. Add a few drops of undiluted oil to the ring. Do *not* add oil to the light bulb itself as the oils are flammable.

Aromatherapy during pregnancy
Aromatherapy is helpful for a variety of pregnancy-associated conditions. It can also help to make childbirth a very positive experience. In a recent study, for example, it was found that a group of mothers who received aromatherapy massage during childbirth felt better, experienced lower stress levels and had decreased labour pains compared with a control group that did not receive aromatherapy massage.

The use of aromatherapy during pregnancy is described below by Marion Simpson, practising aromatherapist and Senior Lecturer in Midwifery at the School of Human and Health Sciences, Midwifery Division, University of Huddersfield:

Aromatherapy for pregnancy, labour and puerperium

Aromatherapy offers a pleasant means of relieving stress, pain, and discomfort and can help to alleviate some of the symptoms experienced in certain physiological, pathological and psychological disorders, by the use of natural substances.

However, there are certain essential oils that should not be used during pregnancy. Indeed, certain authors would say no essential oils should be used during pregnancy,[1] as we do not know what effect the oils will have on the developing fetus. Others, such as Tisserand and Balacs, however, argue that there is no justification for restricting essential oil use to certain specified periods during pregnancy.[2] Caution should be exercised throughout the antenatal period with any oils that are potentially hazardous.

If a woman has a history of bleeding or miscarriage then avoidance of those essential oils that possess emmenagogic properties (i.e. stimulating menstrual flow) during the first trimester, and around the time when a period would be expected, is prudent. Essential oils are highly concentrated substances and it is the chemical constituents within them that give the oils their therapeutic properties. It is the interaction of the essential oils within the body that enables them to be used for medicinal purposes, or can render them potentially toxic when misused. Essential oils are fat soluble, and are readily absorbed through the skin and carried to all parts of the body via the circulatory system and the lymphatic system, before being finally eliminated by the body.

Aromatherapy treatments have a psychotherapeutic effect on the body; the aroma of the oils used will influence the psyche, while the absorbed oils work on the tissues and organs, creating and main-

---

[1] GRACE, U. M. (1996). *Aromatherapy for Practitioners*. Saffron Walden: C. W. Daniels Company Limited.
[2] TISSERAND, R. AND BALACS, T. (1995). *Essential Oil Safety: A Guide for Health Care Professionals*. Edinburgh: Churchill Livingstone.

taining harmony throughout the whole body. However, when put into context, there are many substances that, if taken or used inappropriately, could be detrimental to health.

Most of the studies regarding the toxicity of the essential oils have been conducted on animals, and therefore I would question the transferability of the results to humans. If essential oils are used with care and appropriately diluted in a carrier medium then the risk of causing harm to the fetus is minimised, but care still needs to be taken as more research needs to be carried out in this area. Mojoy[1] recommends dilutions of 0.5 per cent, no more, during pregnancy; others state 1-2 per cent. I have found I use varying dilutions from 0.5-2 per cent depending on the individual.

Certain of the essential oils considered safe in pregnancy have phototoxic (light-sensitising) effects; these are mainly the citrus oils. During pregnancy there are raised levels of circulating melanocytic hormone, leading to a potentially increased photosensitivity of the skin. Therefore pregnant women should be advised against direct exposure of the skin to the sun or sun lamps following administration of any of these oils.

The obstetrical history of the mother must always be considered, and a more restrictive use of essential oils should be considered for those who fall into a high risk group. Always seek medical advice if unsure.

Essential oils that I have found to be particularly useful are given in the following table.

Essential oils found to be useful during pregnancy

FIRST 16 WEEKS	
Frankincense—*Boswellia carterii*	Ginger—*Zingiber officinale*
Mandarin—*Citrus nobilis*	Peppermint—*Mentha piperita*

[1] MOJOY, G. (1996). *Aromatherapy for Healing the Spirit*. London: Gaia Books.

16–37 WEEKS, PLUS THE ABOVE

Bergamot—*Citrus bergamia*

Cypress—*Cupressus sempervirens*

Lavender—*Lavendula angustifolia*

Neroli—*Citrus aurantium*

Rosemary—*Rosmarinus officinale*

Sandalwood—*Santalum album.*

Chamomile (Roman)—*Anthemis nobilis*

Geranium—*Pelargonium graveolens*

Lemon—*Citrus limonum*

Patchouli—*Pogostemon patchouli*

Rosewood—*Aniba rosaeodora*

---

37 WEEKS ONWARDS, PLUS ABOVE

Clary sage—*Salvia sclarea*

Rose—*Rosa damascena/otto*

Jasmine—*Jasminum officinale*

Nutmeg—*Myristica fragrans*

POSTNATALLY

Benzoin—*Styrax benzoin*

Geranium—*Pelargonium graveolens*

Peppermint—*Mentha piperita*

Chamomile (Roman)—*Anthemis nobilis*

Lavender—*Lavendula angustifolia*

Rose—*Rose damascena/otto*

Blends that I have found especially useful during pregnancy and childbirth and their method of application are discussed below.

- Massage (M)—use 25–30 ml of carrier oil (not nut based). I tend to use 80 per cent sunflower and 20 per cent calendula with the essential oil in 1 per cent dilution.
- Lotion or cream base (L/C) (fragrance, lanolin and mineral-base free)—dilutions are as above.

- Inhalation (I)—use essential oils on a tissue, in a vaporiser, or directly on the hand.
- In water (W)—add to baths (oils dispersed using bath base, full fat milk or honey), sitz baths, or foot baths.
- Compresses (C)—these can be hot or cold.
- Gel (G)—arnica or aloe vera jelly (minimum 60 per cent aloe vera content) are an effective transport medium.

Antenatally
General relaxing blends include:

- neroli three drops and lavender two drops (M, W);
- neroli three drops and sandalwood three drops (M, W—useful for urinary tract infections);
- rose two drops and frankincense three to four drops (M, W, I—useful for panic attacks, as it calms the breathing);
- rose two drops and ylang-ylang three drops (M, W, I—also slows down the breathing, and is calming).

Fluid retention: Use geranium two drops and rosemary four drops (M, L/C).
NB: Rosemary is not to be used if the woman has any degree of hypertension.

Insomnia: Use sandalwood four drops and lavender two drops (M, W. I).

Indigestion: Use lemon four drops and peppermint two drops (M, L/C, I).

Mood swings: Use bergamot four drops and geranium two drops (M, L/C, I).

Nausea: Use ginger three drops and peppermint three drops (I).

Stretch marks (linea nigra): Use patchouli two drops, frankincense two drops and mandarin two drops, **or** geranium two drops, mandarin two drops and frankincense two drops, in 80 ml of lotion or cream and 20 ml of wheatgerm. Massage into the abdomen, thighs and breasts from 16 weeks of pregnancy, as soon as the 'bump' becomes obvious, twice daily. As the pregnancy advances increase the area massaged.

Varicose veins: Use cypress four drops and geranium two drops (L/C, C, G).

Haemorrhoids: Use cypress two drops, lemon two drops and Roman chamomile two drops (C, G).

Hypertension: Use rosewood six drops (M). Research conducted by McArdle[1] into the treatment of gestational and pregnancy-induced hypertension with rosewood reported some successful cases. Care needs to be taken if the woman is taking drugs to lower blood pressure.

Intranatally—labour
Use lavender 12 drops, clary sage 12 drops and jasmine/rose four drops in 100 ml of carrier oil to help strengthen uterine contractions and give a feeling of well-being (M).

Frankincense, one drop in the palm of the hand or on a tissue, is helpful for calming and hyperventilation.

Nutmeg (two drops) is helpful as an analgesic, applied over the suprapubic and sacral regions (C).
NB: This is not to be used if the mother has had pethidine; this is due to its myristicin constituent. Although no studies have been done with non-oral dosages of myristicin (as in nutmeg essential oil) and pethidine, its safety is uncertain therefore it should not be used.

---

[1] McARDLE, M. (1992). Rosewood in pre-eclampsia. In *International Journal of Aromatherapy*, **4**, 1, 33.

Postnatally

General use: Use lavender two drops, geranium two drops and rose two drops (W).

Sore nipples: Use benzoin four drops, rose three drops and Roman chamomile two drops (C/L).
NB: This must be removed completely before breast feeding.

Mastitis: Use Roman chamomile three drops, peppermint two drops and geranium two drops (C).

As well as the above use of essential oils, general advice regarding diet, exercise, the use of drugs and the importance of stopping smoking are all offered to provide a holistic approach to midwifery care.

The Pregnancy Shop (TPS) (see Useful Addresses, p. 220, for mail order details) supply their own range of essential oils and recommend the following for use during pregnancy.

First three months

Nausea and vomiting: Use grapefruit or spearmint essential oils.

Anxiety: Use chamomile, bergamot, neroli, mandarin, sandalwood.

Constipation: Use mandarin, orange, grapefruit, neroli.

Headache: Use spearmint.

Second trimester

Indigestion: Use chamomile, ginger.

Insomnia: Use chamomile, lavender.

Third trimester

Backache: Use chamomile.

Skin problems: Use tea tree.

Haemorrhoids: Use cypress.

Labour
Use TPS Labour Massage Oil combining rose (to prepare the uterus for labour), petitgrain and lavandin.

Postnatally

Perineal care: Use lavender.

Depression: Use orange, mandarin, neroli, bergamot, geranium, rose, jasmine, sandalwood, ylang-ylang.

Retained placenta: Use lavender, jasmine.

To encourage lactation: Use fennel or dill tea.

Cautions
- If you are unsure whether or not an essential oil is safe for use during pregnancy, always seek advice from a qualified aromatherapist.
- Do not take essential oils internally.
- Before using an essential oil blend on your skin, put a

small amount on a patch of skin and leave it for at least an hour (patch test) to make sure you are not sensitive to it.

- Do not use essential oils if you suffer from high blood pressure or epilepsy, except under specialist advice from a qualified aromatherapist.
- Keep essential oils away from the eyes.
- If you are taking homoeopathic remedies, do not use peppermint, rosemary or lavender essential oils as these may neutralise the homoeopathic effect.
- Essential oils are flammable, so do not put them on an open flame.

BACH FLOWER REMEDIES

Bach flower remedies are homoeopathic preparations in which flower essences are preserved in grape alcohol (brandy). They are designed to help a variety of emotional states including those that can occur during pregnancy.

Flower remedies were devised earlier this century when a homoeopathic doctor, Edward Bach, realised that patients suffering from the same emotional problems benefited from the same homoeopathic treatment, irrespective of the physical symptoms they were suffering. This led him to the belief that physical symptoms were due to underlying emotional stresses which, if not remedied, would inevitably lead to more serious future illness. He classified emotional problems into seven major groups, which he then subdivided into a total of 38 negative or harmful states of mind. For each of these emotional states, he identified a complementary flower essence that could restore emotional balance.

Bach flower remedies are prepared by either infusion or boiling. In the infusion method, flower heads are placed on the surface of a small glass bowl filled with pure spring water. This is left to infuse in direct sunlight for three hours, then the flowers are discarded and the infused spring water preserved in grape alcohol. This resultant solution is called the 'mother tincture', and is further diluted to create the individual stock remedies.

In the boiling method, short lengths of twigs bearing flowers or catkins are boiled in pure spring water for 30 minutes. The plant material is then discarded and the water allowed to cool before being preserved in grape alcohol. The resultant solution is the mother tincture, which again will be further diluted for use.

Stefan Ball, consultant at the Dr Edward Bach Centre, describes how the Bach flower remedies may be helpful during pregnancy:

Bach flower remedies during pregnancy

The Bach flower remedies are 38 flower- and plant-based medicines. They are unusual medicines in that they do not treat physical symptoms, but instead rebalance emotions and treat negative mental states—such as worry, anxiety, despondency and guilt.

The remedies were discovered in the 1920s and 30s by a highly regarded pathologist and bacteriologist called Dr Edward Bach. They are still made today by his successors, who work out of his old home in Oxfordshire, but the remedies are much more than local products. They are now exported to 66 different countries, and are used by millions and millions of people around the world, including many doctors—and midwives.

They are ideal medicines to use during pregnancy. This is because they are very gentle, very safe and very effective. They are made using the non-toxic flowers from different bushes, trees and plants. These are prepared in water, and brandy is added as a preservative. Like homoeopathic medicines they are extremely dilute, so that there is no measurable amount of plant matter left in the bottle by the time you buy it—so you would be able to take a remedy even if you were allergic to the plant used to make it.

Each of the 38 remedies is directed at a specific cluster of negative emotions. The kinds of the remedies that are often used during pregnancy would include the following.

- *Crab Apple*: used to help you feel good about the way you look. Crab Apple is also useful to take during periods of morning sickness, especially if you have a particular dislike of nausea and sickness.
- *Olive*: used for mental and physical tiredness. A couple of drops of Olive can be taken in a glass of water whenever you feel that the effort of carrying around the baby is more than you can cope with.
- *Walnut*: used to help you adjust better to the changes you are going through.
- *Mimulus*: used for fears about giving birth or about the effect the pregnancy is having on you. Mimulus is the remedy for 'known' fears—in other words, fears that have a definite cause you can name.
- *Red Chestnut*: used to ease any exaggerated fears for the welfare of the baby. This is another fear remedy, like Mimulus, but is specifically for people who are anxious not about their own welfare but about the well-being of someone else. If you are anxious about your own *and* your baby's health, then Red Chestnut and Mimulus together might be the answer.

The remedies are available over the counter in most good chemists and health food shops. It might seem that the easiest way to take them is to put two drops from the 'stock bottle' (i.e. the bottle you buy in the shop) on to your tongue. But this does use a lot of remedy up, and is less convenient if you are taking more than one remedy at a time.

It is usually better to take the remedies in water. To do this, put two drops of each selected remedy into a glass of water and sip from the glass until the feelings have passed. You can mix together up to seven remedies at a time.

You can also use this method if you want to take the same remedies over a longer period of time, such as a few days or weeks. However, most people in these circumstances find it more convenient to make up a 'treatment bottle' To do this get an empty 30 ml dropper bottle from the place that you bought the remedies, and put into it two drops of each selected remedy. Again, you can use up to seven different remedies. Top up the bottle with non-fizzy mineral water, and add a teaspoon of brandy if you want to to help the water stay fresh. The dosage from a treatment bottle is to take the remedies four times a day, taking four drops each time. You can take more-frequent doses if you need to.

Probably the most famous of the Bach flower remedies is Rescue Remedy. This is a premixed combination of five remedies (Rock Rose, Impatiens, Clematis, Star of Bethlehem and Cherry Plum) and is used to help at times of crisis. Not surprisingly, it is a popular choice among pregnant women, especially when labour starts. It contains remedies to counteract faintness, shock and loss of self-control, and because it helps you stay on top of the experience you will be able to enjoy it more than you might have expected to. (I know I am a man writing this, so what do I know?—but my wife used Rescue Remedy during the births of our three children, and each time the midwives were impressed by the way she coped. As was I.)

The dosage for Rescue Remedy is the same as the treatment bottle dose: four drops at a time, or four drops in a glass of water and sip as needed. For convenience in the delivery room you might want to add the drops to small bottles of mineral water and sip from those. You can also add Rescue Remedy to cold compresses.

There is no danger of overdosing on the remedies, and they are not habit forming and will not harm your baby or you in any way. Neither do they react with or counteract the effects of other medicines. The only possible warning relates to the brandy that is used to preserve them, but even then the amount of alcohol taken once they have been diluted is extremely small. However, if you have any doubts at all about taking the remedies you should ask your doctor or midwife for advice.

Finally, the remedies can also be a great help after the baby is born. Unaccountable depression could be helped with Mustard, difficulties in adjusting eased with Walnut, and irritability washed away with Impatiens or Beech. Once you have made their acquaintance during your pregnancy you may well find that the remedies become an everyday friend and partner as you and your new baby continue to grow together.

For contact details of the Dr Edward Bach Centre, see Useful Addresses, p. 226. The full list of Bach flower remedies is as follows.

Fear

- Rock Rose (*Helianthemum nummularium*) is for extreme terror, panic, fright and nightmares.
- Mimulus (*Mimulus guttatus*) is for known fears (e.g. phobias), timidity and shyness.
- Cherry Plum (*Prunus cerasifera*) is for fear of losing control, uncontrollable rages, tempers, impulses, and fear of causing harm to oneself or others.
- Aspen (*Populus tremula*) is for vague fears and anxieties of unknown origin, and sense of foreboding, apprehension or impending doom.
- Red Chestnut (*Aesculus carnea*) is for excessive fear or overconcern for others.

Uncertainty and indecision

- Cerato (*Ceratostigma willmottianum*) is for those who doubt their own ability to judge situations or make decisions.
- Scleranthus (*Scleranthus annus*) is for the indecisive and those subject to energy or mood swings.
- Gentian (*Gentianella amarella*) is for the easily discouraged, those who hesitate, are despondent or self-doubting.
- Gorse (*Ulex europaeus*) is for feelings of despair, hopelessness and futility.
- Hornbeam (*Carpinus betulus*) is for 'Monday morning' feelings of not being able to face the day, tiredness, procrastination and those needing inner strength.
- Wild Oat (*Bromus ramosus*) is for those who are dissatisfied in their current lifestyle or career and who cannot decide which alternative path to follow.

Insufficient interest in present circumstances

- Clematis (*Clematis vitalba*) is for those who live more in the future than in the present (escapism), lack of concentration, daydreaming, lack of interest in present circumstances, and out-of-the-body sensations.
- Honeysuckle (*Lonicera caprifolium*) is for those living too much in the past, nostalgia and homesickness.
- Wild Rose (*Rosa canina*) is for apathy, resignation to circumstances and making little effort to improve situations or find happiness.
- Olive (*Olea europaea*) is for total exhaustion, mental or physical, also weariness and sapped vitality, especially during convalescence.
- White Chestnut (*Aesculus hippocastanum*) is for persistent, unwanted thoughts, mental arguments and preoccupation with worry.
- Mustard (*Sinapis arvensis*) is for deep gloom descending for no apparent reason, melancholy and heavy sadness.
- Chestnut Bud (*Aesculus hippocastanum*) is for those who fail to learn from their mistakes.

Loneliness

- Water Violet (*Hottonia palustris*) is for those who prefer to be alone, or are superior, aloof, proud and reserved in attitude, also for those who will advise but do not get personally involved in others' problems.
- Impatiens (*Impatiens glandulifera*) is for those who are quick in thought and action but irritable or impatient, especially with those who are slower.
- Heather (*Calluna vulgaris*) is for excessive talkativeness and those constantly seeking companionship and an ear to listen, also for the self-absorbed who find difficulty in being alone.

Oversensitivity to influences and ideas

- Agrimony (*Agrimonia eupatoria*) is for those not wishing to burden others, covering problems up with a cheerful façade, and for those seeking out company and good times to avoid facing up to their problems.
- Centaury (*Centaurium umbellatum*) is for those who cannot say 'no', also for the subservient, who are anxious to please and easily exploited.
- Walnut (*Juglans regia*) is for stabilising the emotions during periods of transition, e.g. puberty or menopause, also for adjusting to new beginnings or relationships.
- Holly (*Ilex aquifolium*) is for negative feelings, e.g. envy, suspicion, revenge or hatred.

Despondency or despair

- Larch (*Larix decidua*) is for those lacking in self-confidence, who anticipate failure and make little effort to succeed.
- Pine (*Pinus sylvestris*) is for self-reproach, guilt and dissatisfaction with one's own actions, also for those who blame themselves for the misfortunes of others.
- Elm (*Ulmus procera*) is for those who overextend themselves, are overwhelmed or are burdened with responsibilities.
- Sweet Chestnut (*Castanea sativa*) is for those who have reached the limits of their endurance, for deep despair or unbearable anguish.
- Star of Bethlehem (*Ornithogalum umbellatum*) is for mental and emotional stress following traumatic experiences e.g. grief.
- Willow (*Salix vitellina*) is for those who feel they have suffered unjust misfortune, and for resentfulness and bitterness.
- Oak (*Quercus robur*) is for the brave and determined, who

never usually give up despite adversity or illness, but who are losing their strength to fight.

- Crab Apple (*Malus pumila*) is for feelings of shame, unworthiness, uncleanliness, poor self-image or fear of contamination; it helps to detoxify and cleanse.

Overcare for the welfare of others
- Chicory (*Cichorium intybus*) is for those who like to keep their family and friends close by, and find it difficult to allow them to go their own way; also for those who expect dutiful obedience in return for the love they give.
- Vervain (*Verbena officinalis*) is for those with strong opinions, those incensed by injustice, the overenthusiastic or argumentative.
- Vine (*Vitis vinifera*) is for those who are strong willed with a tendency to be ruthless, domineering, dictatorial or inflexible.
- Beech (*Fagus sylvatica*) is for the critical and intolerant, those who seek perfection and are continually finding fault.
- Rock Water (*Aqua petra*) is for those who are overly strict with themselves, or hard taskmasters with a severely disciplined lifestyle.

CHIROPRACTIC

Chiropractic is a mainstream complementary treatment that is widely accepted by the medical profession and, for some problems such as back injuries, is often more effective than orthodox medical treatments. It is based on the belief that poor body alignment and abnormal nerve functioning are a direct cause of ill health. The spinal column is made up of 33 small bones (vertebrae) that surround and protect the spinal cord. The upper 24 vertebrae (cervical, thoracic and lumbar) are separated from each other by pads of cartilage called intervertebral discs. These have a tough, flexible outer case with a soft, jelly-like centre. Intervertebral discs cushion the vertebrae when you move your back, and act as shock absorbers to prevent damage from sudden jolts. When the spinal column becomes misaligned, a nerve may become trapped, compressed or stretched, leading to pain, discomfort or restricted mobility. A misalignment of the joints can occur for many reasons, including poor posture, pregnancy and childbirth.

The word 'chiropractic' is derived from the Greek *cheir*, meaning hand, and *praktikos*, meaning done-by. Chiropractors have a finely tuned sense of touch and literally use their hands to manipulate the spine with rapid, direct yet gentle thrusts to realign muscles, tendons, ligaments and joints. This strengthens the body's nerve supply, corrects poor alignment, eases tension and promotes relaxation. The key to the success of these adjustments is in the speed, dexterity and accuracy with which they are performed.

Gentle chiropractic treatment during pregnancy can help to relieve headache, back and pelvic problems, heartburn and insomnia. It may also make childbirth easier. The first treatment session typically lasts 30–60 minutes, with follow-up sessions taking 15–20 minutes.

Manya McMahon, writing on behalf of the British Chiropractic Association, explains below how chiropractic may be beneficial during pregnancy:

How chiropractic may be beneficial during pregnancy

You don't have to be expecting a baby to know that pregnant mothers suffer a whole range of uncomfortable 'side-effects'. These may be anything from nausea and back pain to constipation, heartburn and fatigue, and most women are only too familiar with the less happy side of being pregnant. In fact, studies show that 50 per cent of women suffer with low back pain during pregnancy.

Chiropractic can often restore the feelings of blooming health and vitality that are supposed to accompany pregnancy. It works on the principle that the nervous system controls every part of the body through the nerves branching off the spinal cord from between each spinal joint. If the joints are not moving properly (as a result of poor posture, stress, accident or other factors) the nerves can be affected and cause discomfort, pain or even disease. Chiropractic involves gentle and specific manipulation of the joints of the spine and limbs, to restore mobility, relieve pressure on nerves and allow the body to heal. No drugs are used, making it an ideal treatment for those who are expecting.

As a baby grows in the womb, the mother's centre of gravity shifts, and the normal curves in her lower back become more extreme. These are likely to affect her posture, and she may find herself leaning slightly backwards to compensate for the added weight in front.

In addition to this, pregnancy triggers hormonal changes that lead to a loosening of ligaments throughout the body. This is of particular importance around the lower back and pelvis, as it allows the baby to pass through the birth canal, and it persists for about three months after birth. Lax ligaments can lead to instability and discomfort in the pelvic area.

The enlargement of the breasts during pregnancy can worsen a tendency to be round shouldered in some mothers, and this may also affect the position of the neck, leading to headaches.

All such changes in posture and pelvic instability may result in pain and discomfort in the pubic area, buttocks, groin, legs, lower back, ribs, neck, head and many other places. Chiropractors use a variety of techniques, specially tailored to suit pregnant women, to treat this pain and discomfort. All are gentle and painless, and they are regularly used to treat patients right up to the time of birth, and again when relief is needed for the stresses and strains of the birth and the handling of a young child.

The first visit to a chiropractor will begin with an in-depth discussion of the patient's symptoms, medical history, lifestyle and posture. She will then be examined using standard neurological and orthopaedic tests, before the chiropractor reports on the findings, gives a diagnosis and begins treatment. The patient will be told how many treatments are likely to be necessary, and over what period of time.

Treatment itself consists of gentle, very specific hand movements, known as adjustments, which are applied to the affected joint in order to restore normal mobility. It may also include other stretching and massage techniques if appropriate. A chiropractor will often also prescribe gentle exercises that will help the patient to strengthen postural muscles, and may offer dietary and lifestyle advice to improve a mother's general fitness as she prepares for the birth, and as she recovers after it.

It is advisable for mothers to return to their chiropractors for a check-up after the birth, to ensure that no further nerve irritation has occurred during or after labour. At this time, chiropractors strongly suggest that the baby is also examined and treated if necessary. This is because birth is one of the greatest physical traumas most of us will experience, and small adjustments early on can make a huge difference to a child's health later.

After the baby's head has engaged, usually during the eighth month of pregnancy, there can be a lot of stress on its head and back as it continues to move within the womb. This stress can increase further during the birth process, particularly if it is prolonged or involves breech presentation or forceps delivery. It may lead to symptoms including colic, prolonged crying, asthma, sleep and feeding problems, breathing difficulties and hyperactivity.

Instead of treating the symptoms with drugs, or assuming that the child will 'grow out of it', the chiropractor will gently adjust a baby's spine to remove the nerve stress. A study in Denmark revealed that, when spinal adjustments were given to 316 infants with colic, 94 per cent were relieved of symptoms within a two week period of treatment.

The chiropractic profession has recently achieved statutory regulation, and the General Chiropractic Council is due to open its Register in June 1999. After two years, once the Register is fully set up, it will be easy to find a reputable chiropractor, since only those accepted for registration will be permitted to call themselves chiropractors.

McTimoney chiropractic

McTimoney chiropractic is a variation of chiropractic developed by John McTimoney (1914–80). The McTimoney philosophy is similar to standard chiropractic in that it focuses on the spine and nervous system, but also considers joints in other parts of the body. During a session, McTimoney chiropractors will use their hands to check and adjust the spine, pelvis, chest, limbs and skull. They use a number of light, swift and dexterous hand movements, unique to McTimoney chiropractic, which include gentle fingertip manipulation to realign joints. They will also usually show you simple exercises that you can do to help yourself.

According to the McTimoney Chiropractic Association the applications during pregnancy are as follows:

Pregnancy is the one time in a woman's life when she not only must be aware of her own health, but the implications on the developing baby inside her. These changes are unparalleled by anything else and encompass many factors, including hormonal, skeletal, ligamental, muscular and tissue changes. McTimoney chiropractic, through its gentle whole body approach, can enhance the health and well-being of both the mother and developing infant. Women are now more aware of their personal health and have a heightened desire to seek answers, and look further for solutions to health problems. These solutions may well be found in chiropractic; for example fatigue, nausea, morning sickness and back ache are common complaints that have in the past been accepted as the 'norm' with pregnancy. McTimoney chiropractic has a pivotal role to play in enhancing the health and well-being of the mother, her pregnancy and her baby. Through regular assessment and adjustments, and by ensuring correct balance within the skeletal system, these symptoms may be kept to a minimum. With regular chiropractic assessments, the pelvic girdle can also be maintained in its optimum position in readiness for the delivery, and to give the baby the best chance of moving into the most natural position for birth.

Women can start receiving chiropractic treatment after the first three months of pregnancy. McTimoney chiropractors work in partnership with their patients, and particularly with women expecting a baby. Wherever possible, the McTimoney chiropractor will also work in co-operation with the general practitioner (GP) and midwife—a letter is normally sent to your doctor informing them of treatment. Simple stretch exercises may be suggested to help maintain muscle tone throughout the pregnancy. Suggestions may be made on posture, and advice given on lifting and carrying to prevent injury, as with the increased weight gain and altered weight distribution the risk of injury can increase. Difficulties in lifting can be due to size, but can often result from lack of knowledge on the correct position.

Although back pain is considered a common feature of pregnancy, chiropractors are often able to offer relief with their subtle adjustments. The number of treatment sessions needed varies from person to person and may involve monthly visits until the last four weeks of pregnancy. Towards the end of pregnancy, misalignments tend to become more frequent owing to either the action of hormones or the increasing size and weight of the baby, and weekly treatments may be advised until the baby is born. Your chiropractor will recommend how soon after birth you should return for treatment to re-establish the natural position of joints, muscles and pelvis, and to keep them functioning well. Babies can also benefit from gentle McTimoney treatment to help overcome the stress of being born.

COLOUR THERAPY

Colour therapy is a complementary technique in which the energies of light waves are used to balance and heal. Natural sunlight contains all the colours of the spectrum: red, orange, yellow, green, blue, indigo and violet. It bathes us in a sea of colour, although this is only obvious when light is split with a prism or atmospheric water to create a rainbow.

Every colour vibrates at its own frequency, as does every living thing—including all the cells in the body. As a result, colour can affect your emotions and well-being. Shades of blue, for example, are restful and can be used to help lower blood pressure, improve sleep and to reduce pain perception, which can be beneficial during childbirth. Exposure to red light, on the other hand, tends to have the opposite effect and can cause blood pressure and feelings of stress to rise as it triggers release of adrenaline. It may therefore be a good idea to avoid surrounding yourself in red during pregnancy and childbirth. Red does have a role to play, however, as magenta is the colour of 'letting go' and used in small amounts can help to free you from some harmful emotions, such as ambivalence about your impending childbirth. Green is the calming colour of nature and can reduce anxiety and tension so that recovery from stress and ill health are quicker where natural settings full of green foliage plants are used.

A colour therapist will use colour vibrations to correct imbalances in the energy vibrations of cells in order to restore the person to wellness during times of stress or ill health. Most therapists use a colour together with its complement (the colour that is opposite in the 'colour wheel' and balancing in its qualities and effects). You may be asked, for example, to choose three out of eight coloured cards to reveal your current emotional and physical state. These colours may be used along with their complementary colours to help balance your vibrational health. A colour therapy device that beams coloured light on to the body is not normally used during pregnancy. Instead, colour therapists will encourage visualisation of colour, channel colour to you through their hands and advise you on which colours to wear and which coloured foods to eat. Coloured drinks can also be used as part of colour therapy. White should be worn underneath therapeutically coloured clothes to filter out unwanted colour vibrations. Colour therapy may also be combined with other holistic therapies such as reflexology, aromatherapy and acupuncture.

Your aura
Everyone is surrounded by an aura of energy, which is made up of seven influences or chakras. Each chakra contains the full spectrum of colour, but one is dominant in each as follows:

- *red*: the root chakra at the base of the spine;
- *orange*: the sacral chakra in the pelvis;

- *yellow*: the solar plexus chakra below the sternum;
- *green*: the heart chakra;
- *blue/turquoise*: the throat chakra;
- *indigo*: the brow chakra;
- *violet*: the crown chakra.

Seeing complementary colours

A colour's complementary vibration can be seen simply by staring at a particular colour for a while, then closing your eyes. The complementary colour will appear as an after-image on the inside of your lids:

- Green is neutral.
- Blue complements red.
- Yellow complements violet.
- Orange complements indigo.

Using colour therapy during pregnancy

Listen to your intuition, which will often let you 'see' the right colours needed to heal your vibrational imbalances.

- Use orange to stimulate emotional, physical and sexual energy as well as lifting your spirits.
- Use yellow to promote clear thinking, self-control, optimism and inner strength, and to resolve unaddressed emotions and feelings.
- Use green for freshness, regeneration and growth. Green is an especially good colour to wear during pregnancy as it helps to neutralise stress and nervous tension, and frees repressed emotions and fears.
- Use blue to lower high blood pressure, calm overexcitement and promote restorative sleep.
- Use turquoise to increase your emotional resistance, boost immunity and protect yourself from the influences and demands of others.

- Use indigo to calm anger, lower stress-related high blood pressure and help overcome addictions.
- Use violet to calm anxiety.

Tips: How to use colour therapy during pregnancy
- Surround yourself with green plants.
- Wear green as often as possible.
- Paint your bedroom with restful blues and greens to induce sleep.
- Colour your living areas with warm sunshine tones for invigoration.
- Wear yellow when you feel the need to boost your inner strength.
- Relax and visualise a healing colour at times of stress— imagine being totally immersed in that colour and breathing it into your body.

CRANIAL OSTEOPATHY

Cranial osteopathy is based on the fact that the joints between the bones of the skull retain slight flexibility, and the belief that the cerebrospinal fluid nourishing the brain and spinal cord pulsates at 6 to 15 times per minute. Practitioners sense the pulsation (known as the cranial rhythmic impulse) with their hands and 'listen' to the inner movements and tensions inside the patient. The skull bones are then gently manipulated to improve circulation of fluid, blood and lymph in the head. Cranial osteopathy may be used during pregnancy to help the same range of conditions as standard osteopathy, such as back and neck pain, headache, insomnia, low spirits and digestive disorders. Cranial osteopathy may also be used on infants to correct distortions caused by a prolonged or difficult birth, and to relieve the irritability and colic that may occur as a result.

Craniosacral therapy is a modern version of cranial osteopathy that involves the gentle laying on of hands and manipulation of both the skull and spine. Practitioners believe that the cranial rhythmic impulse affects every cell in the body owing to the continuity of fluids and tissues. The laying on of hands and manipulation are therefore believed to release inner energy and tensions over a wider area. Most people experiencing craniosacral therapy feel deeply relaxed during the treatment and notice spontaneous unwinding of tension owing to the release of physical and emotional imbalances. It may be helpful for low back pain, headache and stress related to pregnancy.

Many chiropractors and osteopaths also practise these techniques with great success.

CRYSTAL HEALING

Crystal therapy involves placing crystals such as quartz on the body to speed healing. Crystals make up one third of the Earth's crust; they are over 40 million years old, took over 10000 years to form and are believed to be tuned to the magnetic core of the planet. Clear quartz is pure silicon dioxide, which allows all colours of the spectrum to pass through it. Coloured quartz absorbs and reflects certain wavelengths of light owing to minute traces of impurities such as iron (in amethyst) and manganese/titanium (in rose quartz). Smoky quartz is formed when rock crystal is irradiated, while citrine develops when amethyst is subjected to heat.

Crystals resonate at their own individual frequency and can receive, store and transmit energy. When pressure is applied to a quartz crystal this energy is given off in the form of an electric current—the basis of their use in electronics. They help you to 'ground' and heal yourself by balancing and restoring energy levels. Kirlian photography reveals that every crystal has its own energy field. When this interacts with your own body field, it will absorb negative vibrations and restore balance to your system, re-energising you. Crystals can also be used to increase the power of meditation and visualisation and to store positive emotions.

Clear rock crystal—which always takes an hexagonal form—is the most versatile healing crystal because of its regular structure and its sharp point, which allow it to receive and transmit energy efficiently. Those that refract light to produce internal rainbow flashes of colour are especially beautiful and powerful. Double-pointed crystals are even more powerful as they can transmit energy in both directions, or receive and transmit energy simultaneously, but they are rare and difficult to find.

In general, it is important to select crystals that you are particularly drawn to, as the right crystal to help heal your current problem will manifest itself. You can also choose particular types of crystal that are known to help heal particular symptoms. As in colour therapy (see p. 95), different-coloured crystals are associated with each of the seven energy centres in the body (chakras) as in the following table.

Properties of crystals

COLOUR	ENERGY CENTRE	CRYSTAL	PROPERTIES
Red	Root chakra	e.g. ruby, garnet	Calming, reducing stress and tension; strengthening the spine and legs
Orange	Sacral chakra	e.g. carnelian	Activating emotions and encouraging openness and release; used to treat all urinary and genital problems

COLOUR	ENERGY CENTRE	CRYSTAL	PROPERTIES
Yellow	Solar plexus chakra	e.g. citrine, tiger's eye, topaz	Strengthening vitality and releasing repressed emotions
Green	Heart chakra	e.g. emerald, jade	Encouraging inner peace, self-acceptance and love; boosting immunity; balancing hormones
Blue	Throat chakra	e.g. aquamarine, turquoise	Encouraging self-expression
Indigo	Brow chakra	e.g. blue sapphire, lapis lazuli	Strengthening intuition and heightening awareness; calming and relaxing
Violet	Crown chakra	e.g. amethyst	Deeply calming and relaxing; overcoming insomnia, headache, stress, anxiety and fear

A similar technique—gem essence therapy—uses vibrations from gem stones to relieve emotional problems. Gem stone essences are made by immersing stones in pure water and leaving them to infuse in sunlight. For instance, emerald essence is said to improve memory.

In crystal zone therapy, a crystal may be used as a massage tool to stimulate acupuncture points and reflexes on the hands and feet.

CYMATICS

Cymatics—a term derived from the Greek *kyma*, meaning 'billowing wave'—is a modern alternative therapy that compares the human body to a musical instrument. Sound waves vibrate at different frequencies, as does every cell within the human body, which is surrounded by an electromagnetic energy field. This resonates at its own individual sound frequency, although inaudible to the human ear. In health, our cells vibrate together in harmony, but if these harmonious relationships become disrupted then disease will result. In cymatics, a practitioner uses a machine to pass healing sound waves through the body to restore and reinforce those frequencies that are normally associated with health and well-being. Cymatics can help to reduce many pregnancy-associated conditions, including stress, anxiety, low spirits, high blood pressure and muscle and joint pains, and can also provide pain relief during labour. According to Dr Sir Peter Guy Manners, who founded cymatics, it is:

> Tomorrow's medicine for today's people. Cymatic therapy works hand in hand with the natural process of the body, renewing and revitalising natural healthy bodies—a method of transplant, not of an organ, but of the energy life force that holds and keeps that organ or structure in health and vitality.

HEALING

Spiritual healing—sometimes known as 'hands-on healing' or 'faith healing'—is a widely practised alternative therapy that may safely be used during pregnancy. In spiritual healing the person with healing ability is not considered to be the original source of the healing power, but acts as a clear channel through which the healing energy may pass and be transferred to the

102

patient—usually through the hands. The source of the energy is believed to be of a divine nature, although you do not have to be religious or to 'believe' in order to receive and benefit from the power of healing. The healing energy that is transferred from the healer helps to boost your body's own natural healing mechanisms, which have become depleted. It may prove helpful for a wide range of pregnancy-associated problems, especially those causing pain. The National Federation of Spiritual Healers describe healing as follows:

Spiritual healing is a natural, gentle therapy treating the whole person: mind, body and spirit. It involves the channelling of healing energies through the healer to the client—usually through their hands—and may be performed in the client's presence or at a distance. The healer seeks to supplement the client's depleted energies through 'attunement'—perhaps best described as a combination of empathy and intent—to release the body's own curative powers to deal with stress, illness, injury and recovery in the most effective way.

Clients receiving healing tend to experience sensations of peace and tranquillity, being re-energised or relaxed, 'pins and needles', heat or coolness. Sometimes, pain is also felt to come to the surface and disperse, indicating that the energies are indeed 'going to work'. Healing can be given for any illness, stress or injury as a completely natural therapy that has no side-effects and is complementary to any other medical treatments. It can help a wide range of physical and psychological conditions, sometimes to a remarkable degree; indeed, the medically diagnosed nature of the illness—whether trivial or terminal—appears to be irrelevant to the outcome. As well as relieving pain and restoring function, healing can also improve attitudes, clarity of thought and quality of life.

There is no need for 'faith'. All that is asked of clients is that they relax and 'think well'. The therapist may need to touch certain areas of the body, mainly the head, shoulders or spinal region (but only with prior agreement) and recipients remain clothed throughout. They may also be given guidelines to promote healing between visits.

Spiritual healing is usually helpful in some way. It is unusual for there to be no benefit. Sometimes one treatment is sufficient, but often several are needed and the benefits emerge gradually. In rare cases, clients may feel worse before improving, but this is often a significant part of the healing process, signalling a release of stress that may have gone unrecognised.

There is a growing trend for healing to be given under the supervision of doctors, and clients are always advised to contact their doctors about any conditions that may need medical attention. Healing is officially listed as a therapy recognised by the NHS, and doctors are permitted by the General Medical Council to refer patients to spiritual healing if they wish. NFSH healers may also attend hospital in-patients who request their services.

The NFSH believe that healing should be freely available to all irrespective of their ability to pay, and many healers make no charge for their services. The NFSH is a charitable organisation dependent upon voluntary contributions to cover the cost of its administration and information services, and NFSH centres therefore usually suggest a small donation of £3–£5.

HELLERWORK

Hellerwork is derived from rolfing (see p. 148) and aims to realign the body and rebalance the link between mind and body. It was devised in the late 1970s by Joseph Heller, an engineer who applied the mechanical principles he had learned to the human body to improve health and vitality. Roger Golten, a hellerwork practitioner, describes his use of hellerwork below:

Hellerwork and pregnancy
Hellerwork attempts to integrate the mind, body and spirit using the powerful tools of myofascial (muscle and connective tissue) bodywork, movement and awareness education, and conversation to relate thinking, feeling, attitudes, emotions and beliefs to the person's experience of being in the body. The major results reported by clients of hellerwork include an effortless improvement in posture, a tremendous increase in body awareness and improved breathing, standing, sitting and walking.

Pregnancy is itself a powerful and natural opportunity for the development of body awareness, bringing consciousness into the body through the big changes that take place on the emotional, physical and existential levels. Sometimes problems such as various kinds of back ache and shoulder or neck tension arise during pregnancy, which lead women to seek assistance. Other times there is a general desire to get into as good a shape as possible prior to the birth. Hellerwork can provide focused attention on optimising wellbeing for such an important and demanding event in one's life.

Hellerwork seeks to empower clients to become the 'expert' on their own bodies, so that they are able to take responsibility and get more of what they want out of life, to be the cause of their lives rather than helpless victims of circumstances. During pregnancy this is particularly appropriate, with the tendency for the medicalisation of childbirth, leading to increased interventions that interrupt this natural process.

As the baby grows and increases in weight, there is an inevitable exaggeration in any postural imbalances in the mother's physical structure. Sometimes the posture of hellerwork clients in the early stages of pregnancy (3–5 months) has improved so much that they appear not to be 'showing' quite so much, decreasing potential discomfort. Hellerwork can be an intense experience in terms of experiencing one's own chronic and formerly unconscious tensions, and learning to let go and trust in a powerful process can assist in the preparation for childbirth. The following specific case histories illustrate the range of applications that arise with the kind of attention given during hellerwork.

Ruth Backway, a fellow practitioner, says:

> I have two memories of working with pregnant clients that may be of interest to you. I am a physical therapist and have been a hellerwork practitioner for 15 years. Because of this, I get medically orientated referrals. I also have a practice inside a medical clinic. One case was a woman in her 30s who had a long history of back problems. This was her third pregnancy. The one she had two years previously was very troubled with low back pain and she was put to bed for a week at a time owing to the pain. Structurally, she had an increased lumbar

lordosis (curvature at the base of the spine) and carried her chest in a position so it was bent backward over her pelvis. She also had her right pelvis tipped at the front and almost no movement in her right sacroiliac (pelvic) joint. She wanted to do the hellerwork so she didn't have such a bad time of it this time around. We worked on her during the second trimester. When working on the psoas muscle, I worked in the middle and high on the muscle, not disturbing the lower abdomen on the deep layers. I also used a technique to help right the pelvis and get the sacroiliac joint moving. The hellerwork took care of the other postural stresses on her back, and she had a routine and comfortable pregnancy.

The other case I recall was the wife of my chiropractor whose clinic I work from. She was 40 and pregnant for the fourth time, but it had been 14 years since her last pregnancy. She came in one day with a very pained look on her face. She was in her final two weeks. She complained she couldn't get comfortable—had strong back pain and couldn't stand up or sit down. The pain was centred in her sacroiliac (pelvic) joints and across the sacrum. On testing, the left pelvis was tipped back and the left sacroiliac joint was stuck. I used soft tissue mobilisation to her piriformis muscles and then the technique I mentioned previously to right her pelvis, and the pain went away. The point here was that in the end stages of pregnancy, when things start to get lax, it is easy for the pelvis to slip a bit and this can cause a great deal of pain. Practitioners need to watch for this, and finding a practitioner who has experience in fixing this type of problem can be very useful.

Tom Merrill, a hellerwork practitioner in California, reports:

Pam was one of my two 'models' for the hellerwork training I attended in 1989–90. This was a year long, non-residential program that involved weekly evening classes and one three day weekend class each month. Thus, the bodywork series for the models spanned over a period of ten months. Pam was approximately 5½ months pregnant when she received session one. Thus, session four landed just a couple of weeks before the little one was due. Session five was delayed a week and done at my mentor's home. Performing the inner thigh session just before the birth and then the belly session right after was a perfect fit. All went well and, as best as I can recall, was uneventful throughout the course of the series. A few years later, Pam called up and scheduled a few more sessions as she was carrying again.

Lonny Fox, a hellerwork practitioner and trainer in Canada, says:

I first met my client, Susan, when I was still working with the Victoria Pain Clinic. She was there on one of the clinic's ten day programs recovering from a motor vehicle accident. At the end of her stay she was improving and was referred to me on an out-patient basis. We saw each other for about eight months, as I was supporting her through her return to work, when she came in one day and asked if I would also support her through her second pregnancy. I was both worried and overjoyed at the prospect of working through this pregnancy with her. I knew it was going to be challenging as she was still experiencing both low back and neck pain from her accident. All went well for most of the pregnancy. She was a very motivated client doing her stretches and watching her posture and movement. She also loved the bodywork and was managing to keep up with her job and look after her two-year-old daughter. I was also enjoying working with two people: the one who gave me the verbal feedback and the one who would kick my hand from the inside when she didn't appreciate a stroke. Throughout Susan managed to be very bright and cheerful, happy about the upcoming birth—that is, until very close to what was supposed to be her delivery date. That Wednesday when Susan came in she was very upset and started to cry almost as soon as she sat down. She told me that her first child had been a cesarean section and she had been hoping in her heart for vaginal birth this time. She had just been to her gynaecologist and he had told her that because the baby wasn't 'dropping' into the pelvic bowl he was afraid that she would probably have to have another C-section. We talked about it for a while and then had a closer look at what was happening. There was such a tight band in the abdomen between the scar tissue from the previous C-section and the pubic symphysis that the baby couldn't get through. That coupled with the worry and fear Susan was feeling meant the whole pelvic bowl, like Susan, was literally 'held in suspense' waiting to see what would happen.

We knew we only had one or two sessions until they were going to induce labor so I started with some very detailed work around the old C-section scar and the pubic bone. Interestingly enough, I didn't get anywhere near the internal complaints that I was used to when I worked the abdominal area. It was as if the baby knew what we were doing. Four days later when Susan came back the baby was 'dropping' but would pop right back up to her old spot in the abdomen. It was as though her pelvic floor was acting like a trampoline bouncing the baby right back up so we went on to do two things. We spent an hour and a half releasing the pelvic floor as completely as possible, trying to clear every old knot and holding from the adductors and the pelvic floor area. At the same time we were doing this I knew that Susan loved the old Disney shows and in trying to think of the birth process I remember the time-lapse photography of chrysanthemums opening. I asked her if she had seen those shots and she said she had. I then checked to see if she thought that was what might happen to the cervix as it dilated for the baby to come through. She loved the idea saying that she really couldn't imagine the process until that moment. I got a call the next day to say her baby had 'dropped' and was in the correct place. Shortly after that her waters broke and she gave birth.

One of the most touching moments of my career came when she called to thank me and let me know that not only had she had a vaginal birth but that, as far as she was concerned, the cervix did open like a flower to welcome the baby through.

As you can see, a trained hellerwork practitioner can provide valuable support at any stage of pregnancy: before, during and after the happy event. At the heart of hellerwork is respect for the client, the hellerwork practitioner meeting the client appropriately at the midpoint between what they have to offer in terms of their skills and compassion and what the client is ready or able to receive. Each pregnancy is an unique process, bringing with it its own challenges and circumstances, problems and opportunities. Like a roller-coaster ride, you can't get off halfway through, but you can learn to surrender to the process and enjoy the ride!

Hellerwork can be considered a valuable adjunctive treatment that pregnant women may consider to further their self-empowerment and their ability to manage their own pregnancies.

HERBALISM

Herbalism or phytotherapy—the use of plant extracts for healing—is now widely used and is one of the most exciting areas of medical research. Different parts of different plants are used: roots, stems, flowers, leaves, bark, sap, fruit or seeds depending on which has the highest concentration of active ingredient. Herbal remedies can have powerful effects: between 30 and 40 per cent of prescription drugs are in fact derived from plants. For this reason, it is important that, with a few exceptions, you do not use any medicinal herb during pregnancy unless advised to by a doctor or qualified herbal practitioner. This is especially important during the first three months of pregnancy when your baby's blueprint is being laid down, although ginger, German chamomile or fennel may be used in early pregnancy to relieve morning sickness. In later pregnancy, garlic, cornsilk, psyllium, meadowsweet and lime flower may be used to relieve certain ailments as described below. Raspberry leaf may also be used in preparation for labour.

Other herbs should be avoided during pregnancy unless prescribed by a qualified herbalist as some can stimulate uterine contractions and should never be used during pregnancy, although they may be recommended during childbirth.

The following advice comes from the Register of Chinese Oriental Herbal Medicine:

Pregnancy and Oriental herbal medicine

Pregnancy usually requires no treatment apart from sufficient food and rest. All women who are pregnant nowadays are involved in the orthodox antenatal care system and problems arising in pregnancy can be discussed with the doctor, who can run all the standard checks for complications. It is of course best to avoid taking anything unnecessary during pregnancy, particularly during the first three months. This includes herbs, which should be given the same consideration and caution as anything else taken in pregnancy. However, herbs, unlike chemically based drugs, are made up from the whole plant, which contains the 'active' constituents and also secondary healing agents, which balance the action of the primary ingredients. Treatment should always be sought from a registered herbalist.

Some problems that arise in pregnancy can often be prevented or lessened if treatment is sought prior to conception, if this is possible. Some of the commonly seen problems are better dealt with this way if planning allows. Someone suffering from constipation or irregularity of bowel movements before pregnancy may find that this gets worse during pregnancy. Someone with a weak or troublesome digestion may be the type to suffer more from 'morning sickness' or indigestion than others. Women who suffer from nasal congestion frequently find this gets worse during pregnancy, and this is a problem that herbs can treat well prior to conception, but is harder to treat during pregnancy. Herbs can serve a really useful function when there have been problems with the menstrual cycle, and there are also many herbs that can help the body to prepare for pregnancy. They also have a place postpartum—for example, stimulating milk production in breast-feeding mothers after the birth.

Herbs can also be helpful in aiding conception where this has proved difficult; many can also help the body prepare for pregnancy. Herbs are particularly useful in pregnancy for the minor problems that orthodox medicine cannot treat so safely. They are not meant to be a substitute for orthodox care, but can certainly help to smooth the path of pregnancy where necessary.

Morning sickness is one of the most common problems in early pregnancy, and usually seen between six and 14 weeks. For mild nausea it is often sufficient to eat little and often, and this can frequently be alleviated by eating ginger. The ginger can either be in the form of fresh ginger, which can be added to food and drinks such as herb and fruit teas (or rice water), or if preferred it can be taken in crystallised form or eaten in the form of good quality ginger biscuits.

Liquorice can also be used to settle the digestion. For more severe nausea, often with vomiting, this may require herbal formulae (acupuncture is also very useful for this). There are quite a few herbs that can help, but they need to be prescribed to fit the type of nausea. For mild to moderate nausea they can be helpful as long as the woman takes the herbs during the time of the day when she feels strongest; waiting until nausea strikes often means the herbs go down only to come straight back up again.

Indigestion, constipation, thrush, piles and heartburn are also all common problems and they can benefit greatly from herbal formulae.

As a general rule, herbs are better taken prior to pregnancy where possible, in order to prevent problems from arising, but can be really useful for those minor but irritating problems that can prevent pregnancy being the pleasurable experience it should be.

Ginger

Research shows that ginger is highly effective in treating nausea and vomiting in postoperative patients and those with excessive morning sickness (hyperemesis gravidarum) who had been admitted to hospital. Ginger can help to relieve morning sickness and flatulence, and relax smooth muscles lining the gut to relieve spasm. It is best taken as a herbal tea, as crystallised ginger or as ginger beer, as the fizziness also seems to be beneficial. Ginger capsules are also available but, as they contain a stronger dose, are best taken under the supervision of a qualified practitioner during pregnancy.

German chamomile

German chamomile is a familiar flower that self-seeds in many gardens. A tea made from the flower heads has a soothing, gentle action that helps to relieve a number of pregnancy-associated conditions such as morning sickness, indigestion, abdominal pain due to wind (colic) and flatulence. It also helps to relax tense muscle, relieves irritability and improves the quality of sleep. Sip small quantities throughout the day, but do not drink more than four cups of chamomile tea daily during pregnancy except under the advice of a qualified herbalist.

Fennel
Fennel tea also has a soothing action on the gut and can help to relieve indigestion, distension, flatulence and colic, and is included in some teething and colic remedies for infants. Fennel also has a mild diuretic action and is helpful for cystitis. Drinking fennel tea after delivery helps to stimulate the production of breast milk. Drink no more than two cups of fennel tea daily during pregnancy except under the advice of a qualified herbalist.

Garlic
Garlic is a popular culinary plant that also has powerful medicinal effects. It has been shown to:

- lower high blood pressure;
- decrease blood stickiness, improve circulation and reduce the risk of blood clots;
- reduce the risk of coronary heart disease and stroke;
- reduce harmful blood fat levels;
- reduce blood glucose levels;
- reduce the risk of a dangerous heart rhythm;
- improve blood flow to the brain, improving memory and concentration.

Garlic powder tablets were recently found to reduce the risk of pregnancy-associated high blood pressure (pre-eclampsia) and to improve circulation through the placenta so that growth retardation associated with pre-eclampsia is less of a problem. Garlic has also been shown to boost placental production of factors that stimulate fetal growth. So, by eating garlic regularly during pregnancy, you may help to improve blood flow through the placenta, boost fetal growth and reduce your risk of pre-eclampsia. Garlic also has antiseptic, antibacterial and antiviral properties. It is often used to treat diarrhoea, wind and indigestion, although if raw cloves are eaten excessively they can produce flatulence. Include garlic in your diet regularly. If you develop pre-eclampsia discuss the use of garlic powder tablets with your obstetrician.

Cornsilk

Cornsilk is the name given to the silky strand-like fronds (stamens) found between the head of a ripe sweetcorn and its covering leaves. It has mild diuretic properties and an infusion in water can help mild fluid retention and cystitis during pregnancy. If fluid retention lasts longer than a few days always seek medical advice so your blood pressure can be checked. Drink no more than four cups of cornsilk infusion daily during pregnancy except under the advice of a qualified herbalist.

Psyllium

The seed and husks of psyllium are a safe and effective remedy for constipation and haemorrhoids. The seeds swell when moistened and become gelatinous, while the husks have a high fibre content. These actions combined provide an effective bulking agent to help regulate bowel motions and overcome constipation. Because it absorbs fluid psyllium is also an effective treatment for diarrhoea. As well as softening the motions, it helps to sooth distended haemorrhoids and reduces irritation. Always drink plenty of water after taking psyllium. Take two teaspoons daily with a large glass of water or—if you prefer— soak in cold water or cold tea overnight before taking.

Meadowsweet

Meadowsweet contains a natural pain-relieving substance, salicylic acid, which is related to aspirin but is much more gentle as a result of the other substances found with it. It relieves pain and inflammation while protecting the stomach against irritation. It may be used during pregnancy to relieve heartburn, indigestion, musculoskeletal pains and as a remedy for diarrhoea. Drink no more than two cups of the infusion (tea) daily during pregnancy, except under the advice of a qualified herbalist.

Lime flower

The flowers of the lime or linden tree are used to relieve headache and sinus pain, relieve anxiety and stress and promote restful sleep. Lime flower may be recommended where high blood pressure is linked with anxiety and stress. It also reduces nasal secretions and is helpful for cold symptoms. Drink no more than three cups of the infusion daily, except under the advice of a qualified herbalist.

Raspberry leaf

Raspberry leaf, taken in the form of tea or tablets, helps to soften the neck of the womb in preparation for delivery, and is recommended daily during the last eight weeks of pregnancy. It should not be taken during early pregnancy. Anecdotal evidence suggests that raspberry leaf extracts reduce the duration and pain of childbirth. Mothers who have taken it often say their contractions were relatively pain free and their baby was born within just a few hours of labour starting. It is thought to work by strengthening the longitudinal muscles of the uterus to increase the force of uterine contractions.

HOMOEOPATHY

Homoeopathy is one of the most popular complementary treatments during pregnancy as it has a great potential for doing good with little or no risk of harm. Homoeopathic medicine is based on the belief that natural substances can stimulate the body's own healing powers to relieve the symptoms and signs of illness. Natural substances are selected which, if used at full strength, would produce symptoms in a healthy person similar to those it is designed to treat. In minuscule homoeopathic doses, however, the opposite effect occurs and symptoms improve. This is the first principle of homoeopathy: that 'like cures like'.

The second major principle of homoeopathy is that increasing the dilution of a solution has the effect of increasing its potency, that is: 'less cures more'. By diluting noxious substances many millions of times, their healing properties are enhanced while their undesirable side-effects are lost.

Homoeopathic remedies are so dilute they are measured on a centesimal scale, in which one part of the mother tincture is diluted with 99 parts of alcohol. This process may be repeated many times: dilutions of 100^{-6} are described as potencies of 6c, dilutions of 100^{-30} are written as a potency of 30c, etc. To illustrate just how diluted these substances are, a dilution of 12c (100^{-12}) is comparable to a pinch of salt dissolved in the same volume of water as the Atlantic Ocean. (A decimal scale may also be used, in which one part of mother tincture is added to nine of alcohol to produce a one in ten dilution; this is designated by the suffix 'x'.)

The way in which homoeopathy works is not fully understood. It is thought to have a dynamic action that boosts your body's own healing power. The principles that 'like cures like' and 'less cures more' are difficult concepts to accept, yet convincing trials have shown that homoeopathy is significantly better than placebo in treating many chronic (long-term) conditions including hayfever, asthma and rheumatoid arthritis.

Homoeopathic remedies should ideally be taken on their own, without eating or drinking for at least 30 minutes before or after. Tablets should also be taken without handling; tip them into the lid of the container, or on to a teaspoon to transfer them to your mouth. Then suck or chew them; don't swallow them whole.

Homoeopathic remedies may be prescribed by a medically trained homoeopathic doctor on the normal NHS prescription form and dispensed by homoeopathic pharmacists for the usual prescription charge or exemptions. Alternatively, you can consult a private homoeopathic practitioner or buy remedies direct from the pharmacist.

Although it is best to see a trained homoeopath who can assess your constitutional type, personality, lifestyle, family background, likes and dislikes as well as your symptoms before deciding which treatment is right for you, remedies can be self-chosen according to your symptoms. In most cases, you should start with a 6c potency. Treatment may be taken two or three times a day for up to a week. If partial relief occurs but the symptoms return once you stop taking the remedy, you can increase the effect by taking a 30c potency. Some practitioners recommend that homoeopathic remedies are taken for up to ten days.

Occasionally, symptoms initially get worse before they get better, especially if you are using homoeopathy alone. This is known as aggravation. Although it is uncommon, try to persevere as it is a good sign that the remedy is working. After completing a course of homoeopathy, you will usually feel much better in yourself, with a greatly improved sense of well-being that lets you cope with any remaining symptoms in a more positive way.

If, after taking the remedies for the time stated, there is no obvious improvement, consult a practitioner to select a remedy that is more suited to you.

NB: When taking homoeopathic remedies, avoid drinking strong tea or coffee if possible as these may interfere with the effect. Similarly, you should avoid using the essential oils of lavender, rosemary and peppermint.

Homoeopathic treatments are prescribed according to your symptoms rather than any particular disease, so they are effective for treating a variety of pregnancy-related problems, as described below by Trisha Longworth, a privately practising homoeopath:

Homoeopathy in pregnancy and childbirth

Our bodies go through many changes during pregnancy, and the healing power is especially active at this time. This makes it an ideal time to build up the health of the mother and her growing baby. Many mothers have doubts over the use of conventional drugs in pregnancy, and turn to homoeopathic remedies because only a minute amount of the active ingredient is used in a specially prepared form. This makes the remedies completely safe, gentle and very effective. Homoeopathic remedies cannot cause side-effects to either the mother or baby, and are completely non-addictive.

Morning sickness is often troublesome during the first few months of pregnancy, usually in the morning when the stomach is empty, although it may occur at any time of day. The traditional cure of eating a dry biscuit before getting up is well worth trying. If the sickness is severe it is worth asking the advice of your homoeopath, but in milder cases Ipecacuanha, Nux vomica, Pulsatilla, Symphoricarcpus or Sepia may help.

Constipation can often be helped by a change of diet, making sure you are getting plenty of fresh fruit and vegetables. Taking iron pills in pregnancy isn't always a good idea, as they can cause constipation and black stools. It is better to increase your intake of iron-rich foods as the baby may deplete your own supply (see p. 32). If anaemia is a problem then a course of Ferrum phosphoricum 6x tissue salts will strengthen the blood.

There are remedies that deal with complications during the birth, such as retained placenta, ineffectual contractions, prolonged labour, uterine haemorrhage, etc., but they need to be prescribed by an experienced homoeopath. The best way to avoid these problems is to have homoeopathic treatment throughout pregnancy. However, there is a lot you can do for yourself. Arnica 6c taken twice a day in the last month will tone up the uterus and prepare the muscles for the birth. Because Arnica is so effective for shock and bruising, it prepares the baby's head for the journey through the birth canal, and minimises the effect of birth trauma, so the baby can settle more easily into its new world. For the mother, Arnica helps prevent uterine haemorrhage as the placenta sheds away from the lining of the womb. Arnica can be taken in the 30c potency every hour during the birth, and three times a day for a few days after the labour. If you have an episiotomy, or if you tear, try bathing the wound with a few drops of Hypercal (Hypericum and Calendula officinalis) tincture in warm water, and healing will take place very quickly. Hypercal is good for sore nipples and nappy rash as well.

Morning sickness

The Society of Homoeopaths has produced an excellent leaflet, 'Homoeopathy in Pregnancy and Childbirth', which includes the following advice on how to select the best remedy for your morning sickness:

Sepia: This is for intermittent nausea that is worse in the mornings and worse for the smell or thought of food, with an empty, sinking feeling in the stomach, which is temporarily relieved by eating, feelings of apathy, exhaustion and heaviness, but oddly is better for vigorous exercise. Indifferent or cross with children and partner.

Pulsatilla: This is for nausea (with little vomiting) that is worse after eating and drinking, and better in the fresh air and for company; where the person feels generally weepy, moody and is better for being comforted.

118

Nux vomica: This is for nausea with retching that is relieved by vomiting, sour belching, retching, indigestion and heartburn; there may be a sensation that there is a knot in the stomach. The person feels very irritable.

Ipecacuanha: This is for constant, deathly nausea with empty belching and retching. Vomiting is difficult and provides no relief from the nausea. The tongue looks clean.

Other homoeopathic remedies recommended by other practitioners for treating morning sickness include:

Cocculus: This is for light-haired women who are sensitive, romantic and easily overstressed by sleepless nights. They feel dull, lethargic, irritable and weak with lack of concentration and headaches. They suffer from nausea at the thought of food and often experience vertigo.

Tabacum: This can help where nausea is continuous, unrelieved and accompanied by a faint sinking feeling in the stomach. The person feels better in the cold.

Cravings

Dr Peter Webb, author of *Homoeopathy for Midwives (and All Pregnant Women)*, recommends the following remedies for those craving certain types of food. Starting with 30c potency, take one dose every time you experience the craving:

Homoeopathic remedies for craving in pregnancy

CRAVING	REMEDY
Beer, brandy, chocolate or cigarettes	Nux vomica
Caffeine	Angostura vera
Eggs	Calcarea carbonica

CRAVING	REMEDY
Fat	Acid nitricum
Ice-cream	Phosphorus
Oysters	Lachesis
Raw food, refined sugar or whisky	Sulphur
Salt	Natrum muriaticum or phosphorus (depending on your constitutional type)
Smoked foods	Causticum
Strange foods (e.g. soil, coal)	Lyssin
Sweet foods	Argentum nitricum or China or Lycopodium (depending on your constitutional type)
Vinegar	Sepia
Wine	Phosphorus or Sulphur depending on your constitutional type)

Homoeopathic remedies may also be taken for a number of pregnancy-associated problems such as colic, constipation, haemorrhoids, cramps, fainting, palpitations, phlebitis, varicose veins, heavy legs, swollen hands, ankles and feet, skin changes, back ache, emotional problems and sleep difficulties. Consult a trained homoeopathic practitioner, or one of the books mentioned in the Further Reading section, p. 218.

Other homoeopathic remedies for pregnancy
The following remedies are widely recommended to treat common pregnancy-related conditions. Full instructions on how they should be taken may be obtained from a registered practitioner or one of the books by Dr Peter Webb (see Further Reading, p. 218).

Homoeopathic remedies for common problems in pregnancy

PROBLEM	SYMPTOMS	REMEDY
Anaemia	Restless and avoids eating eggs	Ferrum metallicum
	Weak, flushes easily yet looks pale	Ferrum phosphoricum
Heartburn	With flatulence and regurgitation	Asafoetida
	With flatulence upwards and downwards	Carbo vegetabilis
	Overweight, with burning tip of tongue	Capsicum
Discharge	Thick, yellow ropy discharge	Hydrastis
	Smelly discharge that stains darkly	Kreosotum
	Prickling discharge	Nitricum acidum
	Bland, non-irritant discharge	Pulsatillum
	Jelly-like discharge	Sepia
Thrush	Copious, irritant, itchy discharge	Helonias
	Candida unresponsive to treatment	Candida albicans
Constipation	Due to weakness of expulsion	Alumina metallicum
	With frequent unsuccessful urges to defaecate	Nux vomica
	For a stool that partially voids then retreats	Silicea

PROBLEM	SYMPTOMS	REMEDY
Haemorrhoids	With sharp shooting pains up the back	Aesculus
	With feelings of a full rectum	Nux vomica
	With itching and burning	Paeonia
	With bleeding, itching and burning plus painless diarrhoea in the morning	Sulphur
Back ache	Lower back pain that radiates to both hips	Kali carbonicum
	Low back pain relieved by firm pressure	Natrum muriaticum
	Back ache worse on starting to move	Rhus toxicodendron
Braxton–Hicks contractions	Uterine contractions towards the end of pregnancy	Cimicifuga
Pain relief during labour	Pain causing red face and moaning, with irrational behaviour	Belladonna

Caulophyllum in preparation for labour

Dr Peter Webb recommends that, at the 37th week of pregnancy, women should start taking the homoeopathic remedy Caulophyllum (blue cohosh) at the 30c potency twice a week (but not on consecutive days) until labour starts. He says 'It makes for an easier labour by strengthening uterine muscular activity and softening the neck of the womb. This means that the baby descends more quickly, reducing the need for episiotomy, forceps and caesarean section.' Caulphyllum can also be used where labour is delayed and for after-pains.

Dr Webb also recommends having the 30c strengths of

Arnica (leopard's bane) and Hypericum (St John's wort) with you at the end of pregnancy to take as soon as labour becomes established: 'The Arnica will reduce blood loss and bruising, and will also stop a precipitate labour. The Hypericum will help heal any vulval damage and, in the unlikely event of a episiotomy, it will help skin healing. In the even more unlikely event of forceps delivery, it will help reduce any sacral pain and, if a caesarean section is needed, will help skin healing.' He continues: 'Staphysagria (stavesacre) should be taken on the 4th postpartum day. It will help the woman adjust to any disappointments she may be feeling if her birth plan didn't follow her wishes, and prevent "post-partum blues". It will also help heal the urethra should catheterisation have taken place during delivery.'

For further information on the use of homoeopathy in pregnancy, contact one of the homoeopathic associations detailed in the Useful Addresses section (p. 230), or one of the books listed in the Further Reading section (p. 218).

HYDROTHERAPY

Hydrotherapy is the use of water in healing. It encompasses a variety of different techniques, including bathing in essential oils, mineral solutions, seaweed extracts (thalassotherapy), mud, peat, spas and sea water.

Temperature plays an important role in hydrotherapy. Cold baths stimulate the metabolism, warm water is used during floatation therapy, hot water to soothe musculoskeletal aches and pains, and steam rooms for cleansing and relaxation. In general, you should use a hydrotherapy technique only under supervision when you are expecting a baby as some forms of treatment should not be used during pregnancy. It is also important not to bathe in water of too extreme a temperature. There is some evidence that too-hot baths may harm the developing baby. It is therefore important to stick to temperatures that are comfortably warm (29–36 °C/84–97 °F), neither too hot nor too cold. Do not get up from the bath too quickly or you may feel faint. It is also important to avoid using a jacuzzi when you are pregnant as this is potentially harmful if bubbles are forced into the vagina.

The simplest way to use hydrotherapy is to review your use of the bath or shower at home and improve the therapeutic and relaxing effects by bathing in a room lit by candlelight and carefully selected aromatherapy oils at the end of a tiring day.

- Add a small sachet (250 g) of Dead Sea salts to a warm bath and relax for 20 minutes. Then wrap yourself in a warm towel, and lie on a bed in a warm room for a deeply relaxing experience. (**NB: Do not get the salts in the eyes. Cover cuts or grazes with petroleum jelly or they will sting**).
- Add diluted neroli oil to a bath of warm water and relax for 15 minutes for general relaxation.
- For morning sickness, add diluted ginger essential oil (or 28 g (1 oz) powdered ginger root) to your bath water.

HYPNOTHERAPY

Hypnotherapy is a complementary therapy that many women have found helpful during pregnancy. Leila Hart, an accredited clinical hypnotherapist, describes hypnotherapy below and how it can help you prepare for childbirth:

Hypnotherapy

Your body responds directly to the messages you send it. With hypnotherapy, you can access the message centre, put in the programmes you want, release the blockages and begin the healing process.

Hypnosis is a natural state of deep relaxation when the door to the subconscious mind (your 'computer program') is open and free to accept new positive messages and to release old, unwanted ones. It allows you to access powerful resources and to make healthy changes in a gentle and safe manner. During a hypnotherapy session, the client is fully in control and can hear everything that is said, so can accept or reject any suggestion given. Positive and sometimes rapid changes can occur in many areas, including: unwanted behaviours and habits, health problems, relationships, phobias and panic attacks, weight control, smoking, stress, lack of confidence, obsessive–compulsive disorders, blocked creativity, pain control and much more.

With hypnotherapy, you:

- learn to create a body/mind control room and to master the controls;
- release unwanted negative messages that create problems and 'dis-ease';
- give your body a chance to work as it was meant to;
- gently and efficiently take back control of your life.

For more serious ailments and deep-seated problems, 'cell hypnotherapy' can be used, working directly with the cells of the body to promote a healing response, by releasing the blockages and causes of the problem at the same time. This is done with the agreement of the client's doctor if she is receiving medical help.

A session lasts between an hour and an hour and a half, and the number of visits needed varies for each person.

Hypnotherapy and childbirth

Hypnotherapy can help to prepare you for childbirth. It can produce a sense of well-being and comfort, induce a deep feeling of peace and reduce pain and tension. Greater muscle control can be achieved and recovery from childbirth is often much faster than usual. Hypnotherapy and self-hypnosis can be used in conjunction with regular natural childbirth techniques, and incorporate deep breathing and visualisation for maximum benefit to both mother and baby. Hypnotherapy can help to make the whole experience a more joyful one, giving the mother greater control over her body and her feelings. An experienced hypnotherapist can assist in the release of deep-seated fears or negative imprints from the subconscious mind so that these imprints no longer trigger off unwanted feelings or behaviours. This is done in a safe and gentle way and is always with the client's permission. A positive trigger (maybe a word or finger movement) can be set up in the hypnotherapy session so that the client can use this to induce a rapid state of relaxation. And self-hypnosis can be taught so that the client can work on herself at home and during labour and delivery. This therapy is gentle and healing and can be used to transform unwanted feelings and behaviours. The client is in control throughout the session.

You can also use gentle self-hypnosis to help overcome anxieties or to achieve relaxation. The following exercise will help:

1 Relax in a warm, quiet, dimly lit room where you will not be disturbed.
2 Sit in a comfortable chair with the phone turned off.
3 Take three deep breaths and imagine a soft, golden light flowing over your body as you breathe out, melting away all stress and relaxing your whole body.
4 Imagine walking down ten very safe steps into a beautiful room. In the room is a full length mirror in which you always look perfect—vibrant and happy and in perfect health. Walk to the mirror and enjoy your reflection.
5 Double doors in the room open on to a wonderful garden, where the sun is gently shining. There are banks of flowers of all colours, trees, and maybe a pond or fountain. Spend time in the garden and let all stress and tension fade away.
6 Explore this peaceful place or just sit and enjoy the sounds of the water and birds. Notice how clear everything looks and how serene you feel.
7 When you are ready, count up from one to ten, and open your eyes on the count of ten feeling refreshed and rested.

IRIDOLOGY

Iridology is a form of diagnosis in which problems with the body systems are recognised through changes in the eyes. Janet Spence describes below how iridology may be useful during pregnancy:

Iridology is a safe, painless, non-intrusive form of diagnosis. Through studying the iris under magnification, inherited genetic weaknesses (and strengths) can be detected, along with tendencies towards certain organ/system dysfunctions. Each part of the iris relates to a particular area of the body, and is as unique to the individual as a fingerprint. Iridology is not a new science; it was used by Hippocrates and Philostatus and iris markings have been left by the Babylonians dating back to 1000 BC.

The iris is made up of connective tissues, containing approximately 28 000 nerve endings, all of which are connected to the brain. In this way, the brain receives continual information regarding organ functions and records these messages in iris markings. These genetic markings, passing from parent to child, give an overall blueprint of the constitution and can point out weakness, often several years before symptoms or discomfort become apparent. In this way, the root causes of illness can be more accurately recognised and the appropriate treatment easier to ascertain.

There are three constitutional types:

- lymphatic: blue, blue-green, grey;
- haematogenic: dark brown;
- mixed biliary: hazel, light brown.

These basic groups are broken down into subgroups before the iris is studied more closely for organ markings.

Iridology can reveal how well the digestive system is functioning and whether nutrients are being properly absorbed. There may be low levels of hydrochloric acid (which is often more prevalent in people with blood group A), which in turn may lead to a greater tendency towards anaemia. If this is spotted early in pregnancy then sensible dietary adjustments can be made, which may mean additional iron supplementation is not necessary. Sluggish liver function and kidney detoxification can all be recognised and, therefore, the appropriate treatments more easily identified. These are just a few indications of how iridology can be a useful tool for preventative health care before, during and after pregnancy.

The natural state of pregnancy is not discernible in the iris, but the physiological changes that can ensue are. A slightly displaced fetus can put pressure on internal organs (e.g. the bladder) leading to discomfort. The inability of the bladder to drain fully could then lead to a greater tendency towards a urinary tract infection. Research shows that changes occur in the pupil as a result of faulty nerve impulses stemming from the brain or spinal cord. The skilled iridologist can, by examining the pupil, determine the area of the spine affected. Poor joint alignment (subluxation) to the lumbar vertebrae 3 and 4 can result in uterine, bladder and urinary problems, lower back ache (sciatica or lumbago) and knee joint problems. Lumbar 5 subluxation can lead to poor leg circulation and swelling of the extremities. Subluxation in the sacral vertebrae (1 to 5) leads to poor bowel elimination, pelvic misalignment and impaired lymphatic drainage. Even a slight tilt or rotation of the pelvic girdle may result in a prolonged labour or tendency towards breeched birth, and so early diagnoses can be very beneficial.

Gentle manipulation may be considered to re-establish the correct blood and nerve supply as necessary.

KINESIOLOGY

Kinesiology is based on the belief that muscle groups are related to internal organs, glands and the circulation. The way muscles and reflexes respond to gentle pressure pinpoints imbalances in body function and energy flow. Problems such as food allergy can also be diagnosed by assessing muscle resistance when, for example, a particular food is held against the jaw or placed under the tongue. Fingertip massage of pressure points is also used to stimulate the circulation and correct imbalances found.

Brian Butler, President of the Association of Systematic Kinesiology, describes how this alternative therapy can help during pregnancy:

Diagnosis is the hardest thing that a doctor or therapist has to do. The simple tests of kinesiology avoid guesswork. The client's body supplies the answer and reveals what it needs to become free of aches, pains and other miseries. Authentic kinesiology (pronounced kin-easy-ology), or AK for short, is one of the most exciting health care discoveries this century for the promotion of better health. The practitioner pushes gently on arms and legs, rubs or massages points that need it, offers nutritional support and suggests lifestyle changes. Most people feel much better even after the first session. Most typical conditions are 90 per cent resolved in three to six visits with client co-operation. Wise people continue to go monthly for maintenance. Of course, only properly trained therapists will give the best results. Regular holistic balancing stimulates self-healing, reduces the possibility of serious illness, enhances health, well-being and longevity and helps to ensure a trouble-free pregnancy.

A mother-to-be is a complete person made up of four clearly defined areas:

- mental/emotional;
- biochemical and nutritional;
- structural and postural;
- energy or 'life force'.

For optimum health, each of these areas needs to be in balance whilst the baby is developing in the womb. AK is a simple, safe and powerful self-help method to help achieve optimum health.

Mental/emotional
A mother-to-be has to have mental strength and emotional resilience. She needs to be calm, tranquil and happy during her pregnancy, certain in the knowledge that her unborn baby will pick up on and reflect her emotional state. It has been established that the unborn child can hear; and responds both to the moods of the mother and also to the sounds and stimuli that the mother is affected by. AK offers many ways to help achieve a calm, contented approach to life. One is called the 'emotional stress release' technique and simply involves using a normal gesture in a specific way. This helps emotional 'strung-out' feelings to drift away in two or three minutes so that anxieties and fears melt away under your own fingertips. A small book explaining how to do this is available from the Association of Systematic Kinesiology (see Useful Addresses, p. 232).

129

Biochemical and nutritional

Although it is not recommended that the expectant mother should 'eat for two', the baby is being formed from the mother's own nutritional resources. Eating correctly for health is vital during pregnancy.

It is well known that having a baby depletes the mother's reserves of nutrients, particularly minerals. It is often suggested that it takes a year or more to recoup what the body has lost. A skilled kinesiologist can help greatly in this regard, using a simple non-intrusive form of muscle testing to determine which minerals and vitamins you may be short of. This is not something it is good to leave to guesswork. The wonderful thing about kinesiology is that it can discover subclinical needs for nutrients long before any deficiency symptoms might appear. This is crucial if conditions like osteoporosis are to be avoided in later life.

Millions now suffer from food allergies and sensitivities. The chances are that if you have sensitivities you will not be aware of them. Regrettably, many babies are born with some degree of reactivity to certain foods. They can even react to the mother's milk if she is not eating foods that are appropriate for her. A visit to a kinesiologist may help avoid this. Muscle testing can find which foods are best for the mother, and which may need to be eliminated to solve her food sensitivities and allergies.

Weaning is also a crucial time for babies, as if they are given inappropriate foods before the digestive system can properly digest them, this can lead to rashes, catarrh and other problems.

Well documented are the poisonous effects of both alcohol and smoking, which affect the unborn child to some degree. If you need to give these up and need some support, kinesiology may help.

Structural and postural

A kinesiologist can give you some real help in this area. Having a baby involves intense muscular activity and it is important that your muscles are in optimum balance for childbirth. A few 'balancing' sessions can greatly assist you to achieve this. You will also benefit from some gentle but thorough daily exercise throughout the nine months. Moderate exercise is of paramount importance for overall health. As the pregnancy progresses, it puts some strain on certain muscle groups and can affect the posture. Strengthening these muscles with AK techniques can be a very positive help as the time of birth approaches.

Energy or life force
Being 'tired all the time' is now an accepted syndrome. This does not have to happen. Kinesiological balancing can gently remove energy blocks and release your natural zest for life all through your pregnancy and beyond.

KIRLIAN PHOTOGRAPHY

Kirlian photography is based on the scientific fact that the body generates electrostatic and electromagnetic fields. The quality of these electrical fields can be photographed and analysed using a Kirlian image. This is achieved by placing a part of the body—usually the hands and/or feet—on a photographic plate that emits a high voltage, high frequency electric signal producing a slight buzzing sensation. The way your field interacts with this can be captured on film as an interference pattern. The shape and intensity of the images obtained can reveal energy imbalances between the two sides of the body. The energy images can also be related to the acupuncture meridians. A technique known as 'body logic' may be used to help overcome areas of tension that may be causing ill health. Kirlian photography has not been found to have adverse effects during pregnancy.

Rosemary Steele, of the Institute of Kirlian Photographers, describes the use of Kirlian photography below:

Kirlian photography is not a therapy but an adjunct to diagnosis. The electronic image can be used for a variety of purposes. The majority of applications relate to monitoring the progress of a treatment—the image showing the changes in the energy flow of the patient. It is comparative rather than absolute.

131

Acupuncturists may use a Kirlian image of the tips of the fingers and toes to corroborate their findings when taking pulses, and to give a visual history. Blood analysis can also be done with this process.

Stress management is a further application of the information provided by the image. Body logic is the name of a simple stress management technique which is used along with the electronic image of the hands. Taking Kirlian images before and after treatment provides corroboration of areas that are stressed, and has enlarged our understanding of which areas of the hand change when different parts of the body relax.

I have worked with pregnant women suffering back ache during pregnancy. Frequently, the imbalances that showed in the Kirlian image resolved using the body logic technique and the back ache lessened considerably. It is useful for clients to see the visual corroboration of the changes and to take the image with them as a reminder of how simple it is to help themselves.

If Kirlian photography highlights the cause of a problem during pregnancy, you may be referred to a doctor or a complementary practitioner for treatment.

MASSAGE

Message is one of the oldest complementary therapies. It involves the healing power of touch and forms the basis of many other alternative therapies including acupressure, aromatherapy and shiatsu. A variety of massage strokes—usually with the hands—are used to stimulate the soft tissues of the body: rubbing, drumming, kneading, wringing, friction strokes and deep pressure. In shiatsu, a Japanese form of massage, practitioners may also use their forearms, elbows, and sometimes even their knees or feet as well as their fingers, thumbs and palms to stimulate pressure points on the skin.
NB: Firm, vigorous or deep pressure should not be applied to the abdomen or lower back during pregnancy.

Massage is very relaxing and also seems to stimulate release of the body's natural painkillers to relieve pain and lift a depressed mood. It also helps to develop muscles and can help to prepare a woman for childbirth, especially one who leads a sedentary life and has not exercised much during her pregnancy. As well as encouraging general relaxation, massage is helpful for easing muscle tension, anxiety, circulatory problems, high blood pressure, back ache, insomnia, low spirits and stress during pregnancy and is also beneficial during labour. According to the London College of Massage:

research shows that massaging oil into the perineum (area between the vagina and rectum) daily for six weeks before term helps to soften and elasticise the tissues so that tearing and episiotomy are less likely. In one study of 29 mothers who massaged the perineum and 26 who did not, episiotomy or second-degree tearing occurred in only 48 per cent of those massaging compared with 77 per cent in those who did not. Use lavender and geranium essential oils diluted with wheatgerm oil, and massage daily for five to ten minutes starting six weeks before your baby is due. The procedure is best carried out following a warm bath to increase circulation and soften tissues, and with an empty bladder. Use a mirror so you can see you are applying the oils to the perineum and the posterior vaginal wall, paying special attention to any scar tissue from previous deliveries. The oil is made up using a base oil of wheatgerm. Two index fingers should be gently inserted two inches into the vagina, pressing down towards the rectum. The massage movement is in a 'U'. This helps the tissues to relax and stretch very quickly. The vagina should also be stretched open for 20 seconds to feel the tingling or burning process associated with the head crowning.

According to the Massage Therapy Institute of Great Britain:

During labour, massage helps to relieve pain by stimulating the body to produce some of its own pain-relieving chemicals, called endorphins. As a result, massage can reduce the need for pain relief during labour. During the first stage of labour, massaging the shoulders and upper and lower spine can help relaxation, while massage that starts at the top of the body and moves down to the feet can help to release energy and accelerate labour. Pressing deeply with the thumbs into the centre of each buttock can help to relieve lower back pain, as can applying a deep, firm pressure on the sacrum with the heel of one hand. In the second stage, massaging inside the thighs will help, while massaging almond oil into the perineum helps it to stretch and become more elastic. This can reduce the need for an episiotomy. During the first few weeks after childbirth, a daily shoulder, neck and back massage will help the new mother to sleep and also renew her energy levels and improve her physical and mental health.

Gentle massage can be carried out by your partner and helps him to participate in the pregnancy in a much closer way. The abdomen should generally be avoided except for the lightest of strokes.

How to give your pregnancy partner a gentle massage
1 Make sure the room is warm and quiet. Soft candlelight and slow, relaxing background music will help to set the right atmosphere.
2 Ask your partner to lie on a large bath towel in a comfortable position. When lying on her back, it helps to place cushions under her knees to reduce the curve of the lower back. By around the fifth month of pregnancy, it is best to lie sideways rather than on the back or front, or to sit

in a reclining position. Cover her with another large towel. The London College of Massage recommend that, when performing back massage, get her to sit forward over a straight-backed chair, leaning on a cushion. For head, neck or foot massage, it is advisable to use a bean bag or cushions with the legs and arms supported. These positions can also be used in labour, with lower back massage performed leaning on the bed while standing, squatting or supported by the wall.

3   If using an aromatherapy oil, make sure you have selected one that is safe to use in pregnancy and that it is diluted properly (see Aromatherapy, p. 72).

4   Warm the massage oil or lotion by placing the bottle in a bowl of comfortably hot water. Alternatively, rub some oil in your hands to warm it before using. If adding extra oil during the massage, warm it before it comes into contact with the recipient's skin.

5   Move the covering towel to expose each area of the body as you start to work on it, then re-cover it before moving on to the next area.

6   It is important to use only gentle stroking movements, especially over the abdomen, and to avoid all percussion, heavy or deep pressure.

7   Use long, flowing, simple strokes that follow body contours, and warm the skin. Keep movements flowing and rhythmic with one hand in contact with the body at all times. As a general rule, stroke towards the heart from whichever part of the body you are working on.

8   Don't forget to massage the arms, hands and feet as well as the back, legs and abdomen.

In many cultures, it is traditional for a woman to receive a daily full body massage, including deep massage of the abdomen, to help her body return to normal after birth. Deep abdominal massage should be avoided for at least a month after having a caesarean, however.

Babies can also benefit from a regular massage. The healing power of touch means that babies who are massaged regularly are more active, fall asleep better and gain more weight than do unmassaged babies—as well as being better tempered, more sociable and less likely to cry. Premature babies who were massaged and gently stroked for fifteen minutes, four times a day, were found to thrive better, put on weight 50 per cent faster and develop improved co-ordination and ability to learn compared with babies who were not touched and massaged.

- Only start to massage your baby when he or she is in good health and has passed the six week health check.
- Wash your hands thoroughly before you start and remove any jewellery and your watch.
- Play some quiet, relaxing music. Show your baby lots of love and affection during the massage and talk or sing quietly throughout, maintaining eye contact as much as possible.
- Make sure the room is warm, wrap your naked baby in a fluffy towel and place him or her on a soft changing mat on the floor.
- Pour a little baby oil or lotion into your hands and rub them together to warm them.
- Gently stroke your baby's chest using sweeping, gliding motions that are firm enough not to tickle but gentle enough not to hurt. You can also make small circular motions with your thumbs.
- Repeat the massage on the arms, tummy, legs and back. Circular clockwise massage around the navel can help to relieve colic.
- Finish the massage by stroking your baby softly and smoothly down the back with one hand following the other.
- Be careful holding your baby afterwards as the skin will be slippery.

Some babies get upset during their first massage. If so, wrap your baby in the towel and cuddle him close. Try again another day. Special classes to show you baby massage techniques are available in many areas—ask your health visitor or midwife.

NATUROPATHY

Naturopathy is an holistic alternative therapy based on the belief that the body can heal itself, given the right conditions. Naturopathy can help you maintain a healthy pregnancy as well as addressing any pregnancy-associated problems that may arise, aiming to identify the underlying cause of illness rather than merely relieving the symptoms. A naturopath will focus on maintaining a balance between the body's biochemistry, its structure and the emotions, and may recommend a variety of treatment options including dietary changes, vitamins, minerals, biochemic tissue salts, herbal remedies, hydrotherapy, massage, reflexology, relaxation techniques and sometimes manipulation. Many are also trained in homoeopathy, herbalism, iridology, osteopathy, chiropractic or psychotherapy.

A healthy lifestyle, with plenty of fresh air, rest, relaxation, sleep and adequate mineral water intake, is important, along with reduced exposure to pollution and a positive mental attitude. Skin brushing, water sprays or friction rubs are often recommended to stimulate skin function and to boost the circulation.

Dietary approaches that are recommended for general health as well as during pregnancy include following a wholefood, high fibre—and preferably organic—diet that concentrates on fresh foods that are as raw as possible. A naturopathic diet is low in salt and fat, high in fibre and antioxidants, and contains plenty of nuts, seeds, grains and pulses for protein. If your symptoms suggest an allergy, you may be advised to avoid certain foods such as wheat or dairy products, and advised on which other foods to eat, or which supplements to take, to replenish the nutrients contained in these foods. If you are stressed and anxious, you may be advised to avoid caffeine.

For morning sickness, a naturopath will recommend eating little and often and avoiding fatty foods. Digestive problems and recurrent candida infections, for example, may stem from lack of friendly bacteria such as lactobacilli in the gut and vagina. You may therefore be advised to eat live 'bio' yoghurt (or take *Acidophilus* supplements) to improve your intestinal and vaginal health. Fatigue may be addressed with vitamin B supplements, while vitamin E may help to avoid or improve stretch marks (see p. 174).

For constipation, molasses are an effective and harmless laxative; take one to two teaspoons daily.

OSTEOPATHY

Osteopathy is a method of diagnosis and treatment based on the mechanical structure of the body. Gentle manipulation of the joints and soft tissues is used to correct poor alignment, relax muscles, improve body function and restore health. Manipulations used range from gentle massage to sudden, swift mobilisations of joints. Osteopathy is more helpful than orthodox medicine for improving low back pain, especially in pregnancy when analgesic drugs are best avoided. Osteopathy can also help other problems not obviously related to the joints and muscles, such as breathing difficulties, as misalignment of the joints can cause pain or disrupt nerve supply to other vital organs. Correcting these helps to restore the body's ability to heal itself. Osteopathy can help a wide range of pregnancy-related problems including muscle and joint aches and pains, neck problems, headache, dizziness, constipation and abdominal discomfort including after-birth pains.

PRENATAL STIMULATION

One of the newest complementary techniques is prenatal stimulation, which aims to enrich the sensory environment of a
developing baby to help him or her reach their full intellectual
potential. A baby's brain is literally shaped by the stimuli and
nutrients received from the environment. Although this process
starts at conception, many parents start their child's learning
programme only from the time of birth. It is now widely felt
that it is more beneficial to begin one stage earlier—while
your baby's brain is still developing in the womb. There is
increasing evidence that providing your baby with an enriched
prenatal environment helps to stimulate its brain development
and enhance both creativity and ability to learn. It can even
boost the number of brain cells your baby is born with, and
the number of connections they make with neighbouring cells.
By encouraging you to interact with your baby several times
a day, the technique also helps you form a special bond with
with him or her, bringing you even closer after birth.

A prenatal stimulation programme is usually started around
20 to 24 weeks' pregnancy. Aim to stimulate your baby for
no more than two hours per day in total.

Using voice
- Speak regularly to your unborn baby, stroking or patting
  your tummy in a particular way to attract attention before
  you do so, e.g. pat three times regularly on both sides of
  your bump so the baby gets to know when he or she is
  being addressed.
- Tell your baby a favourite story once a day.
- Introduce new stories throughout your pregnancy and tell
  them regularly, in addition to the familiar story you are
  telling every day.
- Get family members to greet your baby as well as you—for

example, when your partner comes home from work in the evening, or a child arrives home from school.

- When talking to family members, tell your baby who they are so the baby has the chance to associate voices with names.
- Some researchers suggest using a speaking tube (e.g. the inside section of a kitchen roll) against the abdomen when talking to your baby so sounds are transmitted in a more focused way.
- Sing to your baby, especially repetitive songs and chants.
- Sing along to your favourite music on the radio.

Using touch

If you wish to stimulate your baby with touch, do so only sparingly for short periods of a few minutes twice a day early on in your pregnancy. During the last six weeks of pregnancy you can massage your baby for slightly longer—up to 15 minutes—and more frequently—up to four times a day. Some things you can try include:

- patting your tummy gently using a regular rhythm;
- regularly and rhythmically stroking your baby while you are talking to him or her;
- rocking your own body to and fro gently, while supporting your abdomen in your arms, or sitting in a rocking chair.

Using light

If you wish to stimulate your baby with light, do so sparingly, only once or twice a day. Some things you can try include:

- holding a torch against your tummy and flashing it on and off slowly, no more than three or four times per day;
- holding a torch against your tummy and flashing it on and off a few times when telling a particular story, singing a particular song or listening to a particular piece of music.

Using BabyPlus

The BabyPlus unit produces a rhythmical, repetitive sound to stimulate your baby through a graded series of 16 different stimulation patterns. Strap on the unit for 45 to 60 minutes twice a day, morning and evening, ideally starting from around 24 weeks of pregnancy. Many mothers have reported that their baby loves the sessions and starts to kick and 'complain' if the BabyPlus session is late. Parents who have used BabyPlus are extremely enthusiastic about the results. They report that their children:

- are relaxed, calm and contented;
- are alert and responsive;
- have good head control at birth;
- have strong backs;
- have incredibly strong grips;
- seem to have heightened senses;
- have excellent memory and concentration skills;
- have long attention spans;
- focus on their parents' faces surprisingly early and can hold their gaze;
- seem very knowing and aware;
- seem empathic and bond closely with family members;
- reach their developmental milestones earlier than expected;
- have remarkable language acquisition skills;
- are sharing and sociable, engaging and responsive;
- are articulate and communicative;
- are sensitive to moods, situations and their surroundings;
- are less fearful of new situations;
- have enhanced creativity;
- are more likely to have a high intelligence, measured in the 125–150 IQ range (the average for the population is 100).

BabyPlus is available by mail order. Call 01787 210777 for details.

Playing music to your baby

You can play music to your baby in the womb using a personal cassette player. This became popular in the 1980s and mothers and researchers alike reported benefits in babies' performances with improvements in understanding, social behaviour, creativity and strength. In the womb, babies seem to synchronise their limb movements to the music they are hearing, almost as if they are jigging along. These limb movement changes last for many minutes. Some parents choose classical music, some pop music and others folk music depending on personal preferences. It is important not to play music that is too complex, however. A simple, repetitive beat seems to work best. The music also needs to be repeated regularly so your baby learns to recognise it. Recent research among three-year-old children who were stimulated with singing and musical training showed they achieved higher marks in standard intelligence tests; similar benefits may occur in the womb, especially with regard to spatial awareness.

- Choose a simple tune that you like and play it once a day.
- Introduce other simple tunes to your baby and play them regularly.
- If you have a musical instrument, play musical scales to your baby so he or she learns to recognise different notes and their relationship to each other.
- Attach a personal cassette recorder to your clothing or a belt around your waist and play your baby music; choose rhythmical, repetitive sounds or chants.

More information is available in my book, *Super Baby* (see Further Reading, p. 219).

QIGONG (CHI KUNG)

Qigong (pronounced 'chee gong') is a Chinese practice/exercise that is sometimes referred to as Chinese yoga. It is a gentle method that uses posture, visualisation or meditation and controlled breathing methods for health and relaxation (amongst other things). Its purpose is to help to channel or build *qi* energy, strengthen the body and internal organs, produce a feeling of lightness and calm the mind. The basic postures are easy to learn and—unlike t'ai chi, which is a more dynamic form of qigong that is also a martial art (see p. 153)—be performed in any order. A recent medical form of qigong, Buqi, uses three vital forces ('vibration force', 'spontaneous movement force' and 'mental force') to prevent, diagnose and cure disease in others. Qigong and Buqi help reduce stress, and improve posture, muscle control and breathing. They can both be used during pregnancy to encourage relaxation and improve muscle tone in preparation for labour.

REFLEXOLOGY

Reflexology is an ancient technique that has links with techniques used in China over the past 5000 years, and also with methods used by the Ancient Egyptians. It is based on the principle that points on the hands and feet—known as reflexes—are related to specific areas or organs in other parts of the body. The feet are most commonly used as the treatment areas, although the hands, back or other areas may also be used. According to the British Reflexology Association:

In the feet, there are reflex areas corresponding to all parts of the body and these areas are arranged in such a way as to form a map of the body on the feet, with the right foot corresponding to the right side of the body, and the left foot to the left side of the body. By having the whole body represented in the feet, the method offers a means of treating the whole body and of treating the body as a whole. This latter point is an important factor of a natural therapy and allows not only symptoms to be

143

treated but also the causes of symptoms. Reflexology can help numerous different disorders such as migraine, sinus problems, hormonal imbalances, breathing disorders, digestive problems, circulatory problems, back problems, tension and stress.

By applying pressure to reflex points, areas of tenderness can be detected that help to pinpoint problems in other parts of the body, including the reproductive tract. By working on these tender spots with tiny pressure movements, nerves are thought to be stimulated that pass messages to distant organs and relieve symptoms. During a session, your feet will be examined then all areas of the foot will be massaged with firm thumb pressure. A full treatment usually lasts 45 to 60 minutes and at the end of each session you will usually feel warm, contented and relaxed.

Reflexology can be used to help maintain health and wellness during pregnancy, and to treat specific pregnancy-associated conditions such as constipation, urinary frequency, low back pain and sciatica. Many midwives also use reflexology to help with pain during labour and to stimulate weak uterine contractions. Some research has suggested that reflexology can shorten the length of an average labour by as much as half, as well as reducing the need for pain relief.

Reflexology can also be useful after childbirth to help relieve urinary tract infections, breast discomfort and difficulty with breast feeding. Ann Gillanders, Principal of the British School of Reflexology, explains as follows:

The benefits of reflexology during pregnancy
Reflexology is a science that deals with the principle that there are reflexes in the feet relating to all the organs, structures and functions of the human body. By applying pressure to minute areas of the feet we are able to stimulate an 'energy flow' through the body from the bases, which are our feet, to the brain. Reflexology relaxes the body,

144

mind and spirit, improves circulation and normalises bodily functions.

In the early stages of pregnancy, morning sickness can be very distressing owing to the hormonal changes that are taking place in the body. Fortunately the symptoms usually subside within the first three months. Thereafter, most mothers feel extremely well until much later in pregnancy when there are often stresses and strains due to the enlargement of the womb. This presses on other organs and may cause various discomforts such as indigestion, constipation and urinary frequency. The later stages of pregnancy may also place stress on the skeleton.

Regular reflexology treatments throughout pregnancy have a beneficial effect on all disorders relating to the digestive system, especially constipation, which can be such an uncomfortable and distressing experience—particularly during the later months. Reflexology will improve muscle tone in the bowel, with quite dramatic effects on constipation. Many patients feel the need to have a bowel action just half an hour after treatment.

Stress on the skeletal structures during pregnancy particularly affects the lumbar spine, which has to bear the weight of the increasing uterus, which, at term, has grown to reach the bottom rib and descends to the lower pelvic area. Ligaments and muscles running alongside the spine stretch to support the extra load, as hormonal changes increase the elasticity of ligaments to allow this to happen. This can lead to musculoskeletal aches and pains, but with regular visits to a reflexologist the discomfort of back ache can be a thing of the past.

Babies seem to love reflexology even while they are still in the womb. Most mothers say that as they have the treatment they can feel their baby kicking. It is recommended that you continue having reflexology right up to and including the early stages of labour.

Practitioners have found that stimulating the reflexology points linked with the pituitary gland in the brain can also stimulate the release of oxytocin to start contractions. Working on reflexes linked with the lumbar spine, pelvic and hip areas can also bring positive results that enable mothers to have better labours.

Reflexology can also be used to bring on childbirth as an alternative to having a baby induced. The British Reflexology Association have heard from several women who were very overdue but were not keen to be induced. Their GPs suggested reflexology and it did seem to work effectively.

REIKI

Reiki is a complementary therapy that is becoming increasingly well known in the UK. Manjit Ubhi, a Reiki Master, describes what it is, and how it can be helpful during pregnancy:

Reiki (pronounced Ray-Key) is a natural method of healing that was discovered by Dr Usui in Japan in the 1800s. Reiki has gained great popularity especially over the last ten years as a simple yet powerful way of bringing both emotional and physical balance and harmony. Much like the 'laying on of hands', reiki involves the placing of hands in a series of positions on the fully clothed body to channel and transmit Universal Energy. All living things resonate energy. We need this life force to keep our physical and emotional bodies balanced and healthy. When we are under stress, ill or feeling down, that energy is vibrating at a diminished rate; reiki will help to speed up the vibrating energy so that the body is resonating at a state of wellness. Reiki not only effects change in the chemical structures of the body by helping to regenerate and rebuild tissues, bones and organs, but also creates equilibrium and balance on a mental level.

In order to practise or receive reiki you do not have to believe in any particular religious or belief system. All that is required of you is that you open yourself to the possibility that Universal Energy can benefit you. A desire to participate in the journey to your own wellness is also required. Being well is not a passive activity; you need to be active in your own healing process. When you receive a reiki treatment you might experience a deep relaxation, a sense of well-being, a release from blocked emotions or physical pain, a deep stillness and a sense of peace.

Reiki energy has an intelligence and wisdom of its own; so, although the healer is carrying out the treatment, the energy will go where it needs to go in order to restore physical and emotional balance. The body is then able to release its potential to heal itself.

Reiki during pregnancy can be a most gentle, yet powerful, non-invasive healing for symptoms such as tiredness, low back pain, morning sickness, mood changes, high blood pressure, stress and emotional disruption experienced both during and after pregnancy.

I remember one mother who was suffering from tiredness and lethargy but also had constipation. Immediately after the healing session she claimed that not only had her tiredness moved on, but also her bowels, and she had to rush off to the toilet! During pregnancy, because of the fear of change, there can be an emotional 'holding on' and this can often result in being unable to 'let-go' of your waste matter.

Reiki does not perform instant miracle cures; however, with regular treatment, which ensures efficient elimination of toxins, better circulation, harmonised energy levels and a stable and confident emotional, mental and spiritual outlook, you might be surprised at your body's ability to heal and maintain itself. Even apprehension and fear experienced in the late stages of pregnancy and the distress at the impending labour can be alleviated through the deep relaxation, balance and confidence gained through reiki healing.

Since pregnancy can be such a major life-changing event it can often resurrect buried emotions, fears or insecurities from the past—so-called 'unfinished business'. Again, reiki can unblock and heal past hurts and wounds in a most graceful and beautiful way. A weekly treatment is recommended, especially around the heart, abdomen and solar plexus areas, to enable the body to handle all the changes and demands that are put upon it.

Reiki can also be used to send healing energy to the baby. I have known babies to give an excited kick as soon as they feel the energy flowing in. By working directly by holding the 'bump' the healer can channel energy that babies will take according to their needs.

The reiki healer is merely a channel, a transmitter; it is your own body's wisdom that knows what it needs to be well and will take the Universal Energy as needed.

147

I remember one mother-to-be who came to me just before a crucial test. She complained the baby must have been picking up her anxiety as it had been disturbed all night. I worked a great deal around the mother's abdominal area and her heart and temple area to calm and destress her. At the end of the session, both mother and baby were relaxed.

Being pregnant can create a sense of being out of control of your own body. Some women have described it as their body not belonging to them any more, from the day to day changes in their bodies to the sense of invasion experienced from medical interventions. Reiki can enable a sense of regaining some of that control, a balance and a grounding so that, even though you are experiencing a life-changing event, you can be in control; no matter what surprises await you, you will be able to meet the challenges with a sense of deep calmness and knowing.

Sadly, acceptance of complementary treatments that can work alongside medical intervention has a long way to go in this country. I am aware of a women's hospital in the Czech Republic where all the doctors and nurses give reiki and the noticeable results are that the births are easier and the mothers more relaxed and in control.

While no one would argue about the benefits of medical intervention for the mother-to-be, it is important that you are able to use complementary techniques, which can be supportive, in working alongside doctors as this can enable you to have a real sense of having some control and participation in the process of your pregnancy.

The cost of a reiki treatment is usually equivalent to the cost of other hands-on therapies like massage. Some healers will offer a discount if you book a number of treatments in advance.

ROLFING

Giselle Genillard is a licensed midwife, a Certified Advance Rolfer, a Touch-in-Parenting Instructor and director of 'Conversations with Women', an organisation 'dedicated to bringing the light back into women's eyes'. Here she describes what rolfing is and how she uses it in pregnancy and afterwards:

Rolfing in the primal year

It was north of the Mexican border and I was about to begin my midwifery training. A wise old man in the desert cautioned me. 'First,' he said, 'don't end up hating men. And second, remember this: in my country the best midwife doesn't deliver the babies. She sits in her doorway and when she sees a pregnant woman, she pulls her in. Then she works her body and moves her about and scolds her a little and when it comes to the birth the real work has already been done.'

I did not remember his words until I saw the difference conscientious prenatal care made to the outcome of the birth and decided to dedicate my time to that pursuit. The wise old man was clearly pointing me in a direction.

In the years that followed my training I practised as a homebirth midwife and a rolfer. Time and experience cemented my belief that there is nothing more important to our nation's health than the time in which the infant is dependent upon his mother. It is during this time, from conception to breast feeding, that the thermostat for health for the rest of our lives is set. Dr Michel Odent, to whose mentorship and inspiration I am indebted, calls this period the 'primal' period. It is then that the immune system, the hormonal system and the primitive brain are formed and reach maturity. Everything that happens at this time has an influence on our basic state of health and after that all we can do is to take care of it the best we can within those parameters.

Rolfing is a system well-suited to these aims. Developed by Ida P. Rolf in the 1940s, it has moved into the forefront of complementary bodily therapies. Based on the principles of yoga and osteopathy, rolfing is designed to work with the distortions to the body caused by the effects of gravity and physical or emotional trauma, all of which tend to distort the structure away from its natural alignment. Over a series of gentle systematic sessions the rolfer slowly stretches and repositions the body's supportive wrappings, called fascia or connective tissue. As the tensions in the fascial system are released and the body is realigned, movement is restored where restriction used to be, pain is alleviated, the physiology improves and general well-being (psychological and emotional) is enhanced. Research on

149

rolfing has been conducted by Valerie Hunt and Wayne Massey at UCLA's Department of Kinesiology and by Cottingham, Porges and Richmond in Maryland. Both studies concluded that rolfing reduces stress, promotes changes in body structure and enhances neurological functioning. It is, indeed, a primary agent for transitions.

And when, except in infancy, does the human body incur so many radical changes as during pregnancy? During the months from conception until birth, the female body gains roughly 10 to 12 kgs, much of it 'centred' around the middle. The endocrine system orchestrates a flow of hormones that provide both for the support of the baby, the relaxing of soft tissue and the emotional lability characteristic of many pregnant women. And whilst the changes are largely around the reproductive system, all systems are affected: the heart increases in size and rate to cope with a 40 per cent increase in blood volume, the respiratory system is charged with an increased demand for oxygen and a decreased space for functioning, the gastrointestinal system is aggravated by hormones and the growing fetus, the urinary system is similarly compromised and the musculoskeletal system is destabilised by joint laxity and a constant and rapidly changing centre of gravity.

Are we surprised, therefore, to find pregnant women complaining of what are termed the 'usual' discomforts of pregnancy—back pain, sciatica, sacro-iliac pain, morning sickness, fatigue, carpal tunnel syndrome, shortness of breath, tendinitis and cramps? And following the birth are the attendant upper back pain, perineal lacerations or C-section recovery, incontinence, pubic symphysis and coccyx pain, and good old exhaustion. These may be 'usual' complaints but are they necessary? Are we able to circumvent these discomforts or do we just have to cope? I know I am not the only person who believes that coping is simply not the best option.

The careful application of the principles of rolfing to the pregnant body have shown that many of the 'usual' complaints of pregnancy are relieved when more space and balance are created through the structure. For example, a primary concept of rolfing is to horizontalise the pelvis. When the pelvis is organised appropriately, the baby is able to settle back against the spine closer to the mother's own centre of gravity rather than tipping the pelvis forward and distressing the lower back and sacral area. Without this constant forward drag, compression of nerves and the tension patterns that held the baby in space are released, resulting in greater ease of movement, less fatigue and definitely less pain.

Another fundamental principle of rolfing is to maximise the capacity of the rib cage to allow the lungs to expand to their fullest and for breathing to be most efficient. As the baby grows he or she starts to take up the space under the diaphragm that God designed for the organs—lungs, liver, stomach and heart. By working the spine and rib cage, the lower ribs are able to fan out to create more space for the baby to ascend and to decompress the vital organs. This has been shown to help heartburn, shortness of breath, costal margin pain and insomnia, and to improve the flow of nutrients to the baby. Decompression of the spinal nerves innervating the stomach may also relieve cases of morning sickness.

Ideally, rolfing sessions would start pre-conception and would continue about once a month through the first year postnatally. This allows for the body's response to the normal adaptations of pregnancy and birth, to help the body open for birth and to come back together afterwards.

Pre-conception, rolfing prepares the 'soil' by improving posture, general mobility and allowing for greater tissue hydration. Rolfing has been known to help in cases of infertility but the evidence is unfortunately so far only anecdotal. It does make logical sense, however, in that the reproductive organs are suspended in an intricate fascial complex that is sensitive to stressors both structural and emotional.

In the first trimester the lumbar spine is less compromised than the thoracic spine which needs to adapt to the rapid growth and sensitivity of the breasts. Nausea and vomiting are other common problems at this time. Emotionally, this is often the time of the greatest volatility as the mother adapts to the sudden flood of hormones and to the implications of the life unfolding in front of her. Sessions during this time might address creating foundations of support and adaptability within the body and without.

In the second trimester many of the problems are caused by structural shifts as the uterus expands out of the pelvic cavity. Unless the posture is well-adapted, the lumbo-sacral and thoraco-lumbar areas are likely to be stressed. At this stage also, the effects of relaxing are beginning to bear on the soft tissue and the residue of accidents or poor posture pre-pregnancy may now be adding their weight to the growing load. Sessions now are more likely to be directly related to previous structural stressors that are now compounded by the growth of the baby.

In the last trimester the baby is rising up under the diaphragm, leaving little room for the stomach or the lungs, and the general increase in weight can make everyday tasks difficult. Our work now is to provide appropriate accommodation for the baby in the mother's body, and to help the mother carry her baby comfortably through the passage into parenthood.

The information imparted both kinaesthetically and verbally through sessions of rolfing will help a woman gain confidence in her body and to choose the birth options best suited to her. I personally do not advocate as a general rule having anyone other than the closest intimates present at the birth, as it has often been demonstrated that difficulties in labour are increased in proportion to the number of people present. I prefer to include information prenatally on ways in which partners may assist the birth in a non-invasive manner.

Sessions *post-partum* are circumscribed firstly by 'the primary maternal preoccupation', commonly known as 'the baby'. Unless there has been a traumatic delivery, the new mother is inclined to focus on the needs of her family rather than herself. Postnatal care is, however, invaluable and provides a long-term investment in the health of all members of the family by assuring that the primary carer is in optimum condition.

One hidden plus of working with a rolfer through the primal period is that it is a unique opportunity for developing a trusting, ongoing relationship with a professional carer through the medium of touch. In this way, the pregnant woman is often able unselfconsciously to address many of the emotional fears and preoccupations that so often accompany the plunge into parenthood.

All practitioners of any modality must be well trained to recognise symptoms of pathology that require referral for medical consultation, and practitioners should be suitably trained to respect the subtleties of pregnancy. Rolfing does not present a risk to a normal pregnancy.

With all its attendant glories, pregnancy is a time of extraordinary potential for transformation. Rolfing can provide a golden opportunity for the pregnant woman to move into parenthood with confidence and ease, and to develop a unique sense of her own personal power and resources.

T'AI CHI CH'UAN

T'ai chi chu'uan—often known simply as t'ai chi—is a form of Chinese movement that is generally practised using slow, graceful movements, focused awareness/visualisation and breathing techniques to achieve total body control, improve the flow of the life energy/force, or *qi*, and calm the mind. It is sometimes described as 'meditation in motion'. However, it is in fact an 'internal' form of martial art that utilises the internal flow of *qi*, together with focusing of the 'mind-intention' and correct body alignment, to have a powerful effect. One of the most popular versions, known as the short form, consists of 24 slow movements and postures that flow effortlessly one into another and can be performed in five to ten minutes. The long form consists of 108 different movements, which takes 20–40 minutes to complete.

Research suggests that t'ai chi can reduce stress and that, as a form of exercise, it can improve breathing efficiency, help with the circulation of blood and lymph, improve balance and counteract osteoporosis.

It is important to learn t'ai chi from a teacher, if possible, although training videos are available. Sessions start with gentle warm-up exercises and are ideally performed every day.

CHAPTER 5

Complementary Therapies for Specific Ailments

The following chapter explores some of the common problems that can affect women during pregnancy, and the complementary techniques that can help. Always follow the advice of your doctor, and let him or her know which therapies you are using—especially where you have found them helpful.

MORNING SICKNESS

Morning sickness with nausea and vomiting affects seven out of ten women during pregnancy. In many ways it is poorly named—for some women it comes on only in the evening, while for others it last virtually 24 hours a day. The exact cause is unknown, but it is thought to be linked with raised levels of oestrogen hormone, low blood sugar or possibly to increased secretion of bile. Another possibility is that it is triggered by increased production of an intestinal hormone. Symptoms tend to start before the sixth week of pregnancy and have usually disappeared by the 14th week, although a few women continue suffering throughout pregnancy.

Excessive morning sickness (hyperemesis) can cause dehydration, severe salt imbalances and a build-up of harmful ketones in the blood as the body turns to burning protein for energy.

154

- Try to eat and drink something before you get out of bed each morning. For example, ask your partner to bring you a cup of tea and a dry cracker, or hot water with lemon and honey.
- Try to eat little and often during the day—avoid greasy foods.
- Keep sipping water or fizzy drinks, even if you can't keep much food down.
- Ginger has excellent antiemetic properties—drink ginger tea, ginger beer, chew crystallised ginger or take ginger tablets.
- Use aromatherapy: place ginger essential oil on a tissue and inhale. Ginger and peppermint can also be combined if you prefer. Other helpful essential oils include grapefruit and spearmint.
- Elasticated acupressure bands that stimulate an acupuncture point (PC6) on the wrist may be beneficial (but see p. 156). These were designed to stop seasickness, but have been shown to help morning sickness in pregnancy, too.
- Homoeopathic remedies: take the following every two hours for up to three days (see p. 118 for more detailed information):
    — Nux vomica 6c for morning sickness, especially if feeling irritable;
    — Pulsatilla 6c for evening sickness, especially if feeling weepy;
    — Ipecacuanha 6c for constant nausea and vomiting;
    — Sepia 6c if you feel nauseated at the sight, thought or smell of food;
    — acupuncture/acupressure have been used to treat early morning sickness for over 4000 years and are highly effective.
- The Bach flower essence Crab Apple is helpful during periods of morning sickness, especially if you have a particular dislike of nausea and sickness.

- Chiropractic can help to overcome nausea and morning sickness.
- Other helpful complementary therapies include: cranial osteopathy, meditation, relaxation exercises, reiki, healing, visualisation and yoga.

If vomiting is severe, always tell your doctor, especially if you feel weak or dizzy, or if your urine becomes dark and scant. These are all possible signs of dehydration.

Acupressure for nausea

Press for five minutes over PC6, situated in the middle of the front of the forearm approximately the breadth of two thumbs above the wrist crease, every two to three hours, or whenever sickness is felt. This has been shown to be helpful. The same effect can be obtained by wearing commercially available wrist bands with a stud pressing on point PC6. These are available from chemists.

Dr Richard Halvorsen

NB: Classical acupuncture says that PC6 should not be used to relieve nausea after the eighth week of pregnancy.

INDIGESTION AND HEARTBURN

Indigestion and heartburn are common symptoms towards the end of pregnancy, when the pregnant uterus expands upwards and starts to press against the stomach. Indigestion (or dyspepsia) are the terms used to describe discomfort or burning felt centrally in the upper abdomen, while heartburn is felt behind the chest bone.

Indigestion is due to irritation or inflammation of the stomach lining by acidic foods or excess acid secretion. In some cases—especially where you have suffered from indigestion before pregnancy, too—indigestion is associated with an infection of the stomach by a bacterium, *Helicobacter pylori*. In the UK, at least 20 per cent of 30-year-old adults and 50 per cent of those over 50 are infected. In some parts of the world up to 90 per cent of 20-year-olds carry the infection. *Helicobacter pylori* is a mobile bacterium that can move around thanks to small whip-like propellers (flagellae). It burrows into the mucous lining of the stomach to avoid stomach acids, leaving a small breach in the wall through which acids can reach the stomach wall. *Helicobacter* then makes a special enzyme, urease, that allows it to coat itself with a small bubble of alkaline ammonia gas. This keeps the bacteria safe from acid attack and at the same time, irritates your stomach wall, making inflammation worse.

One of the commonest causes of heartburn during pregnancy is acid reflux, in which stomach contents reflux up into the oesophagus (the tube connecting the mouth and stomach). Normally, this is prevented by a sphincter muscle, and by downward contractions of muscles in the gut wall. This protective mechanism may fail during pregnancy owing to increased pressure on the stomach. Acid reflux causes hot, burning sensations in the chest that may rise up into the throat. It usually comes on within 30 minutes of eating a meal and may be triggered by eating too much, taking exercise, bending or lying down. Meals containing fat, pastry, chocolate, acidic fruit juices, coffee or alcohol are the commonest culprits.

Several self-help measures will help to control symptoms of indigestion or heartburn:

- Eat little and often throughout the day, rather than having three large meals.
- Eat your food slowly and chew properly. Don't gulp mouthfuls down.

- Stop eating once you feel comfortably full.
- Don't exercise straight after eating.
- Do not eat for at least two hours before going to bed.
- Drink fluids little and often, rather than large quantities at a time.
- Avoid hot, acid, spicy and fatty foods.
- Avoid tea, coffee, acidic fruit juices and alcohol.
- Avoid your own trigger foods, e.g. fresh bread, pastry, onions, red meat, cheese, citrus fruits or tomatoes.
- Avoid stooping, bending or lying down after eating.
- Elevate the head of the bed about 15–20 cm (e.g. put books under the top two legs).
- If symptoms develop, try drinking semi-skimmed milk to neutralise the acid.
- Indigestion tablets or chews based on calcium are safe to take during pregnancy. Avoid those containing aluminium, however. Your pharmacist will advise on which you can take during pregnancy.
- Colloidal silicic acid gel lines the stomach, absorbs toxins and irritants and protects an inflamed stomach lining from self-digestion with stomach acid. It is therefore effective in the treatment of acid indigestion and heartburn and is safe to use in pregnancy.
- Research suggests that honey made from the Manuka, or New Zealand tea tree, contains essential oils, antiseptics and natural antibiotics that can eradicate *Helicobacter* infection. It is effective even when diluted 20 times. Studies show that taking four teaspoons of Manuka honey, four times per day (on an empty stomach), for eight weeks might get rid of the infection without the unpleasant side-effects associated with conventional treatment. (**NB: Do not use this honey treatment if you are diabetic or have abnormal blood sugar levels during pregnancy.**)
- Meadowsweet may be used during pregnancy to relieve heartburn and indigestion. Drink no more than two cups

infusion daily during pregnancy except under the advice of a qualified herbalist. Fennel tea also helps to relieve indigestion.

- Papaya (paw-paw) contains enzymes (e.g. papain) that help the digestive process; try eating one for breakfast every day until symptoms improve.
- Homoeopathy: take 6c strength as often as necessary:
  — for indigestion with flatulence and regurgitation take Asafoetida;
  — for indigestion with burning tongue and thirst take Capsicum;
  — for indigestion with flatulence upwards and downwards take Carbo vegetabilis.
- Acupuncture can be highly effective.
- The Alexander technique can help to relieve digestive problems.
- Aromatherapy: lemon and peppermint together can help indigestion, or alternatively try chamomile or ginger.
- Other complementary treatments that can help to reduce indigestion include chiropractic, cranial osteopathy, healing, qigong, reflexology and reiki.

CONSTIPATION

Constipation is difficulty in passing motions, usually because they are too hard. Most doctors define constipation as passing bowel motions less than twice a week, or straining at the stool for more than 25 per cent of the time. Constipation is a common and distressing feature in pregnancy and results from a combination of progesterone hormone relaxing the smooth muscles lining the bowel, so bowel activity decreases, and from the enlarging womb pressing against the intestines to impede bowel movements. Because bowel contents stay inside you for longer than usual, increased amounts of fluid are then reabsorbed in the colon so motions become harder in consistency. As a result, they may scratch the anal margin during defaecation and cause blood-staining of the toilet paper after voiding. If you are not sure whether bleeding is coming from the rectum or vagina, always seek medical advice. Other factors that can contribute to constipation during pregnancy include poor fibre or fluid intakes and taking iron supplements.

- Follow a wholefood diet containing more brown bread, brown rice, cereals, salads, fresh fruit and vegetables for roughage. Snack on apples, bananas, pears, grapes, dried apricots or figs when hungry, rather than crisps, cakes or biscuits.
- Soak five to six prunes in water or cold tea overnight and eat for breakfast with natural 'bio' yoghurt.
- Add seeds (e.g. sunflower, pumpkin, fenugreek, fennel and linseed) to salads and yoghurt for extra roughage.
- Natural bulking agents (e.g. bran, wheat husks, ispaghula taken with plenty of water) can be bought to increase the volume of bowel motions and soften them by absorbing fluid.
- Herbalism: the seeds and husks of psyllium are a safe and effective remedy for constipation. Molasses are also an effective and harmless laxative. Take one to two teaspoons daily.
- Drink plenty of fluid: at least six glasses of mineral water per day to swell up the dietary fibre and get things moving.
- Try to take more exercise such as walking, swimming or cycling.
- Applying hot and cold compresses to your abdomen can help, especially if followed by an aromatherapy abdominal massage: gently massage your abdomen with diluted oils of ginger or (after the 16th week of pregnancy) lemon or sandalwood. Other helpful aromatherapy essential oils include mandarin, orange, grapefruit or neroli.

- Massage the abdomen in a clockwise direction, starting on the lower left side.
- Herbalism: take garlic tablets at night.
- Homoeopathy: (take every two hours for up to ten doses):
  — for constipation with little desire to open the bowels take Alumina 6c;
  — for constipation with strong urges to open the bowels take Nux vomica 6c;
  — for constipation with large, hard, dry, crumbling motions take Bryonia 6c;
  — for a stool that partially voids then retreats take Silicea 6c.
- Insert a glycerol suppository to help ease motions and reduce straining. Straining can also be reduced by leaning forwards from the hips when opening your bowels.
- Acupuncture can be highly effective.
- Other helpful complementary therapies include: reflexology, osteopathy, reiki and chiropractic.

HAEMORRHOIDS

Haemorrhoids (piles) are dilated varicose veins that form in the rectum and around the anus when valves in the veins that usually prevent back-flow of blood give way under pressure. This is especially likely during later pregnancy when the bulk of the womb presses on pelvic veins to cause congestion. Piles form soft, fleshy lumps that may remain inside the back passage or be visible outside. Swollen veins close to the anal opening are called external haemorrhoids, while those occurring higher up in the anal canal are known as internal haemorrhoids. Symptoms include a constant dragging sensation, and bright red bleeding, which is sometimes copious. Haemorrhoids may also itch—especially if they are prolapsed and produce a mucous discharge. External piles sometimes become hard, intensely painful and dark purple-black in colour if the blood trapped inside them starts to clot (thrombosed pile). This usually resolves spontaneously over two to three weeks, but consulting a doctor, who will anaesthetise the area and gently evacuate the clot through a small incision, brings instant relief. If you suffer from haemorrhoids during pregnancy:

- Eat a mild, non-spicy, high fibre diet and drink plenty of fluids.
- Use glycerol suppositories to ease motions and reduce straining; straining can also be reduced by leaning forwards from the hips when opening the bowels.
- Relieve the pressure of the uterus on your pelvic veins by lying on your left side for 20 minutes every few hours.
- Bath or shower every day using unperfumed soap and finish by spraying the area with cold water.
- Keep the area scrupulously clean to help stop itching. Wash with unscented soap after each bowel motion and pat dry with soft tissue. If necessary, keep dry using a hairdryer set on gentle heat.
- Wear loose cotton underwear, changed at least once a day.
- Avoid talcum powder.
- If you scratch at night, try wearing cotton underwear and even cotton gloves.
- Aromatherapy: after the 16th week of pregnancy try adding one drop of peppermint oil and two drops of chamomile to warm water (in a bidet or large, shallow plastic bowl) and sit in the solution for five or ten minutes. If the area feels sore and burning, you can also add two tablespoons of bicarbonate of soda. Cypress, lemon and Roman chamomile essential oils are another helpful combination.
- Herbal medicine: astringent ointments containing comfrey, horse chestnut or witch hazel are used; horse chestnut also strengthens supporting tissues around the veins. The seeds and husks of psyllium are a safe and effective remedy for constipation and haemorrhoids.

- Homoeopathy (take four times daily for up to five days):
    — for piles with burning, soreness and bursting feelings take Hamamelis virginica 6c;
    — with sharp shooting paints up the back take Aesculus;
    — with feelings of a full rectum take Nux vomica;
    — with itching and burning take Paeonia;
    — for feelings of heat, burning and itching when overheated, bleeding or associated with painless diarrhoea in the morning take Sulphur 6c.
- Acupuncture can also be highly effective.

Haemorrhoids usually resolve quickly after giving birth.

How piles are classified
- First-degree piles: these are confined to the anal canal and bleed only occasionally.
- Second-degree piles: these prolapse on opening the bowel but reduce spontaneously or can be pushed back in, gently.
- Third-degree piles: these persistently prolapse outside the anal canal.

HEADACHE AND MIGRAINE

Headaches can occur during pregnancy as a result of hormonal changes, stress or poor posture causing tension in the neck and scalp muscles. A tension headache feels like a severe, continuous pressure on both sides of the head, which may seem to centre over the top of the skull, over the back of the head or above both eyes. Some tension headaches feel like a tight, constricting band, whereas others are more like a non-specific ache. Migraine is a more serious type of headache that can also be linked with hormonal changes during pregnancy. Migraine is usually felt on only one side of the head, or is definitely worse on one side, and may be accompanied by abdominal symptoms such as loss of appetite, nausea, vomiting, dislike of food, constipation or diarrhoea. One in ten migraine sufferers also experience visual disturbances although, contrary to popular belief, these are relatively uncommon. When they do occur, vision may be distorted with shimmering or flashing lights, strange zig-zag shapes (known as fortification spectra) or blind spots. Both migraine and tension headaches can be brought on by feelings of excess pressure, physical fatigue, lack of sleep, missed meals and stressful emotions such as anger. They may also be triggered by the relief of stress, such as occurs at the end of a long, trying week.

- Look for signs of tension in the way you sit and stand. Try not to stoop when standing or sitting, and concentrate on keeping your back straight, your shoulders square and your abdomen lightly pulled in. This reduces tension by helping you to breathe correctly. The Alexander technique can improve your posture and symptoms.
- Avoid folding your arms tightly and shake your arms and hands regularly to relieve tension in your upper limbs and shoulders.
- Avoid clenching your fists. Hold your hands loose with your palms open and your fingers curled lightly and naturally.
- Avoid clenching or grinding your teeth, which tenses the jaw muscles.
- If you suffer from migraine, try to work out what factors trigger your attacks and, where possible, avoid them.
- Massage: gentle manipulation of muscles in the neck, shoulders and back can help to relax taut muscles and relieve tension headache.
- Acupuncture can be highly effective.
- Herbalism: lime flower blossoms are used to relieve headaches. Drink no more than three cups of infusion or tea daily except under the advice of a qualified herbalist.
- Homoeopathy: it is best to consult a practitioner for an

individual diagnosis and treatment tailored to you. The following treatments are often used at a dose of 10c every ten minutes for up to ten doses:

— for blinding, throbbing or burning headache take Natrum muriatricum or Nux vomica;
— for right-sided headache take Sanguinaria;
— for left-sided headache take Spigelia or Ipecacuanha;
— for tension headache that comes on suddenly and feels like a tight band take Aconite;
— for tension headache that is brought on by emotional stress, with a sharp, severe pain in the side of the head accompanying the tight band sensation, take Ignatia;
— for a tension headache that feels bursting and crushing, with sharp pain brought on by the slightest movement take Byronia;
— for tension headache with muscular spasm and stiffness in the neck take Cimicifuga racemosa.

- Aromatherapy: essential oils that can help a tension headache include peppermint or spearmint and, after the 16th week of pregnancy: chamomile, geranium and lavender.
- Crystal therapy: carry an amethyst with you at all times.
- Other helpful complementary therapies include: chiropractic, osteopathy, cranial osteopathy, craniosacral therapy, cymatics, healing, reflexology and reiki.

ANAEMIA

Anaemia literally means 'lack of blood'; it occurs when the concentration of the red blood pigment, haemoglobin, falls below normal levels. Haemoglobin is found inside red blood cells and carries oxygen around the body.

During pregnancy, the volume of blood in your circulation increases by as much as a third. The commonest form of anaemia is due to lack of iron, which is needed to produce haemoglobin in the body. Overall, an extra 550 mg of iron is needed throughout pregnancy—300 mg for your baby, 50 mg for the placenta and 200 mg to offset the blood lost during childbirth. Iron supplements are no longer given routinely, however, as the body becomes more efficient at absorbing and using iron during pregnancy, and also your losses decrease as menstruation has temporarily ceased. Anaemia can also occur in pregnancy owing to lack of folic acid or vitamin B12.

When anaemia occurs, body tissues may not get enough oxygen for their needs and symptoms of paleness, dizziness, tiredness, lack of energy, shortness of breath on exercise, headache and even palpitations can occur.

A common symptom of iron deficiency during pregnancy is a craving for strange foods such as soil or cola. This is known as pica. If it happens to you during pregnancy, start taking a supplement containing iron immediately. Ask your pharmacist or doctor for advice on dosage. Your doctor may also want to perform a blood test to check your iron stores.

- A healthy intake of iron helps to prevent iron deficiency anaemia (see p. 32).
- Taking a supplement especially formulated for pregnancy that contains iron, folic acid and vitamin B12 will help to reduce the risk of anaemia.
- When eating iron-rich foods, or taking iron supplements, wash them down with orange juice as vitamin C helps to ensure optimum absorption of dietary iron from the intestines.
- Naturopathy: beetroot and beetroot juice are recommended to help build the blood.
- Homoeopathy: take Ferrum metallicum or Ferrum phosphoricum tissue salts 30c, twice daily.
- Diagnostic techniques such as kinesiology, iridology and Kirlian photography may be able to help pinpoint the cause of anaemia.

CRAMP

A cramp is a painful muscular spasm due to excessive contraction of muscle fibres. This is thought to be linked with a build-up of lactic acid. Cramping often occurs during pregnancy as a result of changes in blood flow and metabolism, or lying in an awkward position as muscles are held unusually tense for prolonged periods of time. Cramping usually affects the calf muscle, but any muscle can be affected. Symptoms usually last for only a few seconds or minutes.

The best way to relieve a cramping muscle is to slowly and gently stretch it (e.g. stretch calf muscle by pulling your foot and toes up in the air) or to massage the bunched muscle fibres. Applying a warm compress will increase circulation and help to bring relief.

To help prevent cramps:

- Increase dietary intakes of calcium (e.g. low fat milk, cheese, yoghurt, etc. and dark green leafy vegetables) and magnesium (e.g. nuts, seafood, dairy products, wholegrains and dark green leafy vegetables).
- Take a good vitamin and mineral supplement designed for pregnancy containing calcium, magnesium and vitamin E, amongst others.
- Ensure you are drinking plenty of fluids during the day, especially mineral water.
- Warm up and stretch for at least 15 minutes before starting exercise.
- Start exercising slowly and gradually build up your exertion.
- Improve poor circulation with garlic tablets and omega-3 fish oil supplements designed for pregnancy.
- Consider taking coenzyme Q10, which increases oxygen uptake in muscle cells, especially when circulation is poor.

- Some nutritionists suggest combining one tablespoon of apple cider vinegar and one tablespoon of honey in a glass and drinking it daily.
- Homoeopathy: relieve cramp by sucking Cuprum metallicum 6c slowly.

RESTLESS LEGS

Restless legs—also known as Ekbom's syndrome—is common in pregnancy and has been associated with fatigue, anxiety, stress and lack of iron or folic acid. Symptoms include an unpleasant, creeping sensation in the legs, along with twitching, pins and needles, burning sensations and a sudden, irresistible urge to move your legs, especially when you are trying to drift off to sleep. Moving the legs relieves symptoms fleetingly, then the irresistible urge returns again.

- Take a vitamin and mineral supplement designed for pregnancy that includes iron, folic acid and vitamin E, among others.
- Consider taking coenzyme Q10—a vitamin-like substance that increases oxygen uptake in cells.
- Garlic tablets may help symptoms by improving circulation.
- Just before going to sleep, try placing the feet in cold water for five minutes to help promote sleep.
- Avoid synthetic socks, tights and underwear as these seem to make the condition worse.
- Avoid caffeine, which may make symptoms worse.
- Complementary therapies that may help include chiropractic, osteopathy, healing, hellerwork, reiki, cymatics, aromatherapy, massage and reflexology.
- Diagnostic techniques such as kinesiology, iridology and Kirlian photography may be able to help pinpoint the cause of restless legs.

PANIC ATTACKS

Panic attacks often occur during a first pregnancy, when the process of carrying and delivering a child can seem an overwhelming task and responsibility. Panic attacks are a natural response to stress and are usually triggered by overbreathing, which means that you give out more carbon dioxide—a waste gas. Overbreathing soon makes your blood mildly alkaline, causing symptoms of dizziness, faintness and pins and needles. These symptoms in turn make your sense of panic worse so you continue to overbreathe, giving out even more carbon dioxide and triggering a panic attack.

- When you feel panic rising, say 'stop' quietly to yourself.
- Breathe out deeply, then breathe in slowly to fill your lungs.
- Hold this breath for a count of three, then breathe out gently, letting your tension go.
- Continue to breathe regularly and gently; imagine a candle in front of your face—as you breathe, the flame should flicker but not go out.
- Consciously try to relax so excess tension drains from your muscles.
- If panic continues to rise, cup your hands over your nose and mouth so you breathe back some of the excess carbon dioxide gas you have exhaled. If you are somewhere private, breathe in and out of a paper bag instead.
- If panic rises suddenly, place five drops of Bach Rescue Remedy under your tongue (see p. 86). The Bach flower essence Walnut can also help you adjust better to the changes you are going through.
- Aromatherapy: rose and frankincense together are useful for panic attacks during pregnancy and calm the breathing. Rose plus ylang-ylang is another good calming blend. Other essential oils good for reducing anxiety include

169

chamomile, bergamot, neroli, mandarin or sandalwood.

- Herbalism: lime flower blossoms are used to relieve anxiety. Drink no more than three cups of infusion or tea daily except under the advice of a qualified herbalist.
- Green, blue or violet can be used in colour therapy to reduce anxiety and tension.
- Crystal therapy: carry an orange carnelian, blue sapphire or lapis lazuli with you at all times.
- Hypnotherapy is highly effective in helping to overcome anxiety, phobias and panic attacks.
- Other complementary therapies that can help to reduce anxiety and panic attacks and improve breathing include cymatics, healing, qigong, t'ai chi, reflexology and reiki.
- Diagnostic techniques such as kinesiology, iridology and Kirlian photography may be able to help pinpoint the cause of your panic attacks.

VARICOSE VEINS

Varicose veins are often triggered by pregnancy and are due to an hereditary weakness in valves in the long veins of the leg that allow blood to flow upwards against the pull of gravity. Increased pressure due to the enlarged uterus pressing on the veins draining blood away from the legs can cause these valves to give way. Blood then pools in the superficial veins, which become dilated and twisted. Symptoms of varicose veins include aching and dragging sensations, swelling of the ankles and feet, itching, bleeding and phlebitis—inflammation of a superficial vein due to clotting of poorly circulating blood. Symptoms usually get worse as the day goes on, especially after you have been standing for long periods of time. Sitting down and raising your legs usually brings relief.

- Massage the overlying skin once or twice a day with a moisturising cream (e.g. E45 or Hydromol cream).

- Walk regularly and avoid standing still for very long.
- Put your feet up as often as possible.
- Extracts of horse chestnut may be gently applied to affected areas in the form of cream to help strengthen the fibrous tissue supporting the swollen veins. Do not massage it in as this may lead to inflammation.
- Homoeopathy:
  - — for uncomplicated varicose veins take Arsenicum album 6c, twice a day;
  - — for painful varicose veins take Pulsatilla;
  - — for varicose veins with tired legs take Hamamelis virginica.
- Ask your doctor about wearing support stockings.
- Acupuncture can be highly effective.
- Aromatherapy: cypress and geranium essential oils may be combined in massage lotion and can help after the 16th week of pregnancy.
- Other complementary treatments that can help include: acupressure, massage, healing, reflexology and reiki.

Varicose veins usually improve significantly after delivery.

CYSTITIS

Cystitis is an inflammation of the bladder. There are three main causes: bacterial infection, irritation due to friction (e.g. honeymoon cystitis) and chemical irritation (e.g. due to excessive urine acidity or to bath additives). Cystitis and kidney infections are more common in women generally as their urethra is much shorter. As many as one in two women experience cystitis at some time during their life. This means infection can more easily reach the upper urinary tract. During pregnancy, cystitis becomes more common as a result of altered immunity and the effects of progesterone hormone, which relaxes smooth muscle fibres within the urinary passage

171

so bacteria can pass upwards more easily. Sexual intercourse is another common trigger of cystitis as it can push bacteria into the urethra. Most urinary tract infections are caused by bacteria that usually live in the bowel. Depending on the severity of infection, symptoms may include:

- burning, stinging or discomfort on passing urine;
- having to rush to the loo;
- passing frequent, small amounts of urine;
- low abdominal pain or backache;
- unpleasant smelling, cloudy or blood-stained urine.

As soon as symptoms of cystitis start, drink a pint (600 ml) of water or weak tea, then drink half a pint (300 ml) every 20 minutes for the next three hours if you can. Passing water may sting initially but will get better as you continue to empty the bladder.

Seek medical advice if:

- symptoms last longer than a day or keep recurring;
- your urine is cloudy or stained with blood;
- you develop a fever or uncontrollable shakes, which suggest infection of the kidney (pyelonephritis).

To help prevent cystitis:

- Tilt your pelvis up when sitting on the toilet so the back passage is lower than the urethra.
- After passing water, lean forwards to squeeze out the last few drops of urine.
- Wipe your bottom only from front to back.
- Wash with warm, unperfumed soapy water after every bowel movement and after making love.
- Use only simple toiletries when bathing as sensitivity to some products can cause inflammation of the urethra.
- Always drink at least two litres of fluid per day.
- Herbalism: drinking 300 ml cranberry juice daily has been shown almost to halve the risk of developing cystitis. Cran-

berry extracts are now also available in capsule form for convenience. Fennel tea and cornsilk extracts also have a mild diuretic action and are helpful for cystitis.

- Apply live 'bio' yoghurt containing *Lactobacillus acidophilus* to the urethral entrance; these friendly bacteria can help to combat infection.
- Homoeopathy (take every 30 minutes up to five doses):
  — take Cantharis 6c for burning pains when passing water;
  — take Apis 6c for stinging pains;
  — take Staphysagria 6c for pain due to mechanical irritation (e.g. honeymoon cystitis).
- Aromatherapy: after the 16th week of pregnancy, add diluted oils of lavender or sandalwood to warm water (ideally in a bidet or wide, shallow bowl) and soak the area for ten minutes twice daily.
- Crystal therapy: carry a carnelian with you at all times.
- Other complementary therapies that can help include cymatics, reflexology, reiki and healing.

Those suffering from recurrent cystitis during pregnancy are usually investigated to rule out gestational diabetes, anaemia or anatomical abnormalities of the urinary tract.

STRESS INCONTINENCE

Stress incontinence is the commonest cause of female urinary leakage and can occur either during the end of pregnancy or after childbirth. Despite its name, it is a physical rather than a psychological problem, and is due to weakness of the pelvic floor muscles. This results in sagging of the bladder and places strain on the natural valve mechanisms (sphincters) keeping the bladder and urethral openings closed. A sudden increase in intra-abdominal pressure, as happens during lifting, coughing, laughing, sneezing or running, then results in urine leaking out.

Weakness of the pelvic floor muscles usually results from difficult or repeated childbirth but is also linked with overweight and the final stages of pregnancy. Pelvic floor exercises are designed to strengthen the muscles supporting the bladder neck and can help get you back into shape after delivery. These exercises are also important after having had a caesarean section as the pelvic floor is stretched by the baby's head coming down during the final weeks of pregnancy even though you have not had a vaginal delivery. Interestingly, research suggests that as many as 40 per cent of women lack normal tone in their pelvic floor muscles.

- During early pregnancy, stand with your feet apart and your knees slightly bent. Place your hands on your hips, jut your bottom out and rotate your pelvis slowly in a clockwise direction. Continue rotating your pelvis round to form a complete circle that is as wide as possible. Continue these pelvic gyrations for one to two minutes, then gyrate your pelvis round in an anticlockwise direction for another one to two minutes.
- Throughout pregnancy, pull up the front and back passages tightly as if trying to stop the bowels from opening. Hold tight for a count of four and repeat this every quarter of an hour.
- Pull in the pelvic floor muscles before coughing, sneezing or lifting and avoid standing for long periods of time.
- Swimming, yoga, walking and other keep-fit activities also help to strengthen the pelvic floor muscles.
- Complementary therapies that may help include healing, hellerwork, reiki, cymatics and reflexology.

STRETCH MARKS

Stretch marks occur when tissues are quickly stretched by weight gain, pregnancy or normal rapid growth during teenage years. Some women seem prone to them, while others never seem to get them at all—it all depends on the type of skin you have inherited. Initially, stretch marks acquired during pregnancy will be a marked purple-red colour. They slowly fade with time, however, until they are pale and hardly noticeable.

- Take regular exercise during pregnancy to keep yourself toned.
- Use a good body lotion to keep your skin soft and supple all over—preferably one containing evening primrose oil, vitamin E, or both.
- Massage the abdomen, breasts, hips and thighs daily during later pregnancy with antenatal massage lotion.
- To treat affected areas, add two drops each of rose bulgar, lavender and tangerine aromatherapy essential oils to two tablespoons (30 ml) of wheatgerm oil (which is rich in vitamin E) and massage in. Other suggested aromatherapy blends include: patchouli, frankincense and mandarin, or geranium, mandarin and frankincense (use only after the 16th week of pregnancy).
- Take evening primrose oil (1 g) regularly throughout the pregnancy for essential fatty acids. Anecdotal evidence suggests that evening primrose oil may help to strengthen your skin and reduce the likelihood of stretch marks.

FATIGUE

Tiredness is one of the commonest problems to affect women in both early and late pregnancy. Several different factors play a role, including hormonal and metabolic changes, the fact that half the nutrients you eat are diverted towards your growing baby, your slowly increasing bulk, and the fact that tiredness is one of nature's ways of reminding you to slow down and rest.

- You'll be surprised how much better you will feel if you eat a healthy, wholefood—and preferably organic—diet. Cut out sweet, stodgy, fatty foods and eat more fresh fruit, vegetables and complex carbohydrates such as wholegrain bread, wholemeal pasta and brown rice. Ideally, you need to eat five servings of fruit or veg per day.
- Adequate supplies of vitamins and minerals are essential for a healthy metabolism. If these are in short supply, you will soon feel tired all the time. The B-group vitamins and iron are especially important, so take a supplement designed for pregnancy that includes these amongst others.
- Coenzyme Q10 can improve physical energy levels and reduce fatigue by increasing the uptake of oxygen into cells.
- Take evening primrose and omega-3 fish oil supplements especially designed for pregnancy, which can help to reduce fatigue.
- Rest once or twice a day by lying down for at least half an hour at a time—this is an ideal opportunity to carry out your prenatal stimulation programme (see p. 138).
- Make sure you get enough sleep which is important for rest, repair, rejuvenation and regeneration.
- Take regular, gentle exercise.
- Cut back on caffeine intake or, preferably, avoid it altogether.
- Acupuncture can be highly effective.
- Aromatherapy: oil of lavender helps fatigue and weakness; orange and geranium oils are uplifting.
- The Bach flower essence Olive is helpful for mental and physical tiredness.
- An homoeopath can recommend particular remedies tailored to your symptoms.
- Yoga, meditation and visualisation can increase levels of mental and physical energy.
- The Alexander technique can help to relieve fatigue.
- Chiropractic can be helpful in overcoming fatigue.

- Crystal therapy: carry a yellow citrine, tiger's eye or topaz with you at all times.
- Other complementary therapies that can help to reduce fatigue include cymatics, floatation, healing, hellerwork, reflexology and reiki.
- Diagnostic techniques such as kinesiology, iridology and Kirlian photography may be able to help pinpoint the cause of fatigue.

INSOMNIA

A good night's sleep is vitally important for you and your growing baby. While lying down, your kidneys find it easier to flush excess fluid and wastes from your system, and blood flow to your placenta increases. During sleep also you secrete more hormones involved in the growth, repair and regeneration of your tissues. Even though rest is so important, however, most women have difficulty sleeping during pregnancy—especially in the last few months.

One of the commonest sleep problems is difficulty in getting comfortable. As your womb enlarges, lying on your back interferes with blood flow through the large vessels (aorta and inferior vena cava) connecting the heart to the lower body. As well as affecting the blood supply to your baby, this can lead to fluid retention and also make you feel faint. Lying on your stomach puts pressure on the womb and becomes impossible after the first few months. Your only option is then to lie on your side, although the weight of your stomach can pull you over and make it difficult to relax.

If you are not used to sleeping on your side, start practising in early pregnancy. It helps to use a few extra pillows. Put one behind you so you don't roll on to your back during the night, or get your partner to snuggle up close. Place another pillow between your knees or fold it in half and place it in front of your legs. You can then roll forwards slightly, with your bent upper leg resting on the pillow. This stops you rolling fully on to your front.

Later in pregnancy, when you produce a hormone (relaxin) that softens your ligaments, back ache can be a real nuisance, especially if you are sleeping on a mattress that is too hard or too soft. Special mattresses made from heat and pressure-sensitive viscoelastic polymers naturally mould to your body so you partially sink into them. Support for the natural curves of your back will help, as this reduces the load on your pressure points and helps your muscles and ligaments recover during sleep. Reduction of strain on your pressure points also reduces the number of times you turn during sleep from 50–80 times a night to around 20 times. It allows you to sleep comfortably on your side without needing extra pillows; your hip sinks into the polymer just enough to support your tummy and make your bulge feel almost weightless. When the baby moves, it feels as though it is wriggling in the mattress rather than in you, which is much less likely to disturb your sleep.

- Eat a healthy, wholefood diet and plenty of unrefined, complex carbohydrates (e.g. wholegrain cereals, brown bread, wholewheat pasta, brown rice) plus fruit and vegetables for vitamins and minerals. Avoid hunger as this will make you more alert, but avoid rich, heavy, fatty meals in the evening.
- Avoid substances that interfere with sleep such as caffeine (e.g. coffee, tea, chocolate, colas) and nicotine. A warm, milky drink just before going to bed will help you to relax; hot milk is better than hot chocolate, which contains some caffeine.
- Try to take gentle exercise during the day as active people sleep better.
- Take time to unwind from the stresses of the day before going to bed—read a book, listen to soothing music or have a candle-lit bath.

- Get into a habit by going to bed at a regular time each night and getting up at the same time each morning.
- Set a bedtime routine such as brushing your teeth, bathing and setting the alarm clock to set the mood for sleep.
- Make sure your bed is comfortable, and your bedroom warm, dark and quiet, as noise and excessive cold or heat will keep you awake. A temperature of 18–24 °C (64–75 °F) is ideal.
- If you can't sleep, don't lie there tossing and turning. Get up and read or watch the television for a while. If you are worried about something, write down all the things on your mind and promise yourself you will deal with them in the morning, when you feel fresher. When feeling sleepy, go back to bed and try again.
- Drinking a soothing, herbal tea is often all that's needed for a good night's sleep. Choose ones containing gentle herbs such as lime flower, lemon balm or rosehips. Lime flower blossom tea is especially helpful. Drink no more than three cups of infusion or herb tea daily except under the advice of a qualified herbalist.
- Homoeopathy: Take the 6c remedy half an hour before going to bed and repeat every half hour if necessary, as follows:
  — for an overactive mind take Coffea;
  — for repeated waking that leaves you irritable and unrefreshed take Nux vomica;
  — if you are overtired and can't get comfortable take Arnica;
  — if sleeplessness is due to fear, panic or shock take Aconitum 30c.
- Aromatherapy oils can also induce sleep. Use mandarin oil during the first 16 weeks of pregnancy. Thereafter, you can use lemon, sandalwood, lavender, chamomile or neroli oils. After the 16th week of pregnancy, try placing a herbal pillow filled with dried lavender flowers at the head of your bed.

179

- Acupuncture and acupressure free blockages in the flow of energy (qi) and stimulate release of natural opiate chemicals in the brain that help you relax. They are excellent for relieving insomnia linked with stress. Acupressure is similar, but stimulates acupoints with firm thumb pressure or fingertip massage (e.g. shiatsu).
- Bach flower remedies are homoeopathic infusions of flower essences in brandy. These 38 different essences can treat most negative emotions that lead to difficulty in sleeping. A practitioner will select the one most suited to your state of mind, e.g.:
  — for vague fears and anxieties of unknown origin take Aspen;
  — for feelings of not being able to face the day take Hornbeam;
  — for total physical or mental exhaustion take Olive;
  — for persistent, unwanted thoughts and preoccupation with worry take White Chestnut;
  — for those who blame themselves for the misfortunes of others take Pine;
  — for those who are overly strict with themselves take Rock Water.
- Chiropractors manipulate the spine with rapid, direct thrusts to correct poor alignment. If sleep is difficult because of tension in your neck, shoulder or back pain, a chiropractor can manipulate your back to realign muscles, tendons, ligaments, joints and bones to ease tension and help you to relax. Osteopathy, cranial osteopathy and craniosacral therapy can also help.
- Hypnotherapy will help to uncover subconscious fears and anxieties that are causing stress. Use of suggestion will help you relax, lose your fears and sleep more easily. Suggestions can be taped and replayed when you go to bed.
- All forms of massage are very relaxing. Therapeutic mass-

age is particularly useful in helping sleep problems due to stress and muscle tension, especially when combined with aromatherapy essential oils.

- Meditation is a self-help technique in which the power of concentration is used to control thoughts and calm the body. During meditation you learn to enter a trance-like state that tunes you into your body; some people can lower their pulse and blood pressure at will. Muscular tension drops, blood circulation improves and brain wave patterns change. Meditation often leads to sleep.
- Reflexology before bedtime will help you sleep—ask your partner to learn the technique!
- Yoga is excellent for improving joint suppleness, relieving stress and helping sleep.
- Blue can be used in colour therapy to promote restorative sleep.
- Crystal therapy: carry an amethyst with you at all times.

By choosing one or more of the above remedies, you should soon be enjoying a good night's rest through natural, gentle means. Once your baby is born, you will be able to sleep on your front or back again. For at least the first few months, however, your sleep will be broken by night feeds. Interestingly, if you breast feed, research shows that producing milk hormones help you to sleep better after waking in the night than if you give a bottle feed.

Another excellent tip is to use a Bed-Side-Bed. This cot has an adjustable base and a removable side and acts as an extension to your bed. Your baby sleeps at the same level as you, making it easy to tend your baby in the night without getting out of bed. For more information call 0181-989-8683.

ITCHING SKIN

Pregnancy is a time of rapid production of new cells and itchy skin is common, especially towards the end of pregnancy. This is usually linked with lack of essential fatty acids, which are needed to make healthy, supple cell membranes and are also needed for healthy development of your baby's skin, nervous system and eyes. Unless you eat around 30 g of nuts or seeds per day and 300 g of oily fish per week, your diet is likely to be deficient in these vital building blocks. Increasing your intake of EFAs will quickly help make your skin feel softer, smoother and less itchy. Anecdotal evidence also suggests that evening primrose oil can help to prevent stretch marks. If you develop severe itching during pregnancy, you should always seek medical advice because occasionally it is a sign of liver problems.

- Avoid excess stress.
- Eat more foods rich in essential fatty acids such as nuts, seeds and oily fish (e.g. salmon, sardines, mackerel and herrings).
- Take evening primrose oil supplements (1 g daily).
- Moisturise your body with a lotion containing evening primrose oil.
- After the 16th week of pregnancy, dilute a total of ten drops of aromatherapy essential oils (selected from chamomile, geranium, sandalwood or lavender) to 50 ml carrier oil; apply to affected area twice a day.
- Use aqueous cream as a soap substitute by simply applying to the skin, massaging in lightly then rinsing off.
- For itchy, flaky scalp, wash hair regularly with a shampoo containing tea tree oil.
- Homoeopathy: take 6c four times a day for up to two weeks, as follows:
  — for dry, itchy skin that is worse for heat and washing take Sulphur;

> — for general itching take Kali arsenicum;
> — for intensely itching skin take Anacardium;
> — for intense itching, especially on the scalp, take Oleander.

- Dead Sea salts contain minerals that can help a number of skin problems including itching. Add to the bath water and soak for at least 20 minutes to help you relax.
- Several moisturising bath additives based on almond or soya oil are also available over the counter to soothe itching skin.
- Diagnostic techniques such as kinesiology, iridology and Kirlian photography may be able to help pinpoint the cause of your itching skin.

Lack of essential fatty acids can cause a variety of symptoms including:

- thirst;
- urinary frequency;
- dry, rough, pimply skin;
- itchy skin;
- dry hair;
- dandruff;
- brittle nails;
- lowered immunity with frequent infections.

LOSS OF SEX DRIVE

Sex drive can go up, down or remain the same during pregnancy—every woman, and every pregnancy, is different. Psychological influences play a large part, as does increased blood flow to the genital area, increased lubrication and the fact that orgasm is usually easier to achieve and more intense. If low sex drive occurs, this is often linked with physical exhaustion, especially during the last three months, a time when levels of prolactin—a hormone that switches on breast milk production and switches off sex drive—are increasing.

After childbirth, prolactin levels return to normal, non-pregnant levels within eight days if you choose not to breast feed. Breast feeding—which is by far the healthiest option for both you and your baby (unless you are HIV positive)—causes prolactin levels to stay high for three months so sex drive is inevitably low. After three months, the sex drive usually returns to normal, whether or not you continue to breast feed.

After your baby is born, you can take steps to improve your sex drive. Take:

- multivitamin and mineral supplement (designed for breast feeding if appropriate);
- essential fatty acid supplements (e.g. Efanatal) or evening primrose oil;
- consider taking coenzyme Q10 if you feel lacking in energy;
- homoeopathy: Phosphoricum acidum, Platinum metallicum, Sepia, Staphysagria (especially if you have had a caesarean);
- aromatherapy: jasmine, rose, ylang-ylang, ginger.

If breast feeding, take the herb agnus castus: 500 mg daily. This stimulates milk production and also boosts libido but should not be taken if using the mini-Pill—in which case take oats (oatstraw) instead: one dropperful of fluid extract or tincture two or three times daily.

If not breast feeding, take St John's wort extracts standardised for hypericin: 300–600 mcg hypericin three times daily. This lowers prolactin levels and boosts sex drive (do not use if breast feeding).

For more information, see *Increase Your Sex Drive* by Dr Sarah Brewer (London: Thorsons).

If low sex drive is linked with postnatal depression, you

must seek medical help from your doctor, midwife or health visitor immediately.

HIGH BLOOD PRESSURE

In around one in ten pregnancies, the mother develops high blood pressure, protein in her urine and fluid retention during the second half of pregnancy—a condition known as pre-eclampsia. Research suggests that pre-eclampsia is linked with poor placental size and function, and with lowered activity of some placental enzymes. If left untreated, it can seriously affect the development of the baby and, in some cases, may progress to eclampsia, a potentially life-threatening condition in which fits occur. If you develop high blood pressure during pregnancy, it is important to follow any advice and treatment suggested by your doctor and obstetrician.

- Taking garlic powder tablets during pregnancy seems to improve maternal blood circulation, stimulate growth of the placenta and increase enzyme activity. Scientists are hoping that garlic extracts can be used to treat poor placental function and pre-eclampsia.
- Folic acid supplements may help to protect against high blood pressure and pre-eclampsia during pregnancy as well as protecting against neural tube defects.
- A high calcium diet may help to reduce the risk of high blood pressure and pre-eclampsia during pregnancy as well as reducing the risk of pregnancy-associated osteoporosis.
- Consider taking an antioxidant supplement containing vitamins C and E.
- Follow a low salt diet. Unfortunately, three quarters of dietary salt is 'hidden' in processed foods such as canned products, ready-prepared meals, biscuits, cakes and breakfast cereals. Cut back on salt intake by not adding salt during cooking or at the table, and by avoiding:

185

— obviously salty foods such as crisps, bacon and salted nuts;

— tinned products canned in brine;

— cured, smoked or pickled fish and meats;

— meat pastes and pâtés;

— ready prepared meals;

— packet soups and sauces;

— stock cubes and yeast extracts.

Salt is easily replaced with herbs, spices, lemon or lime juice as it doesn't take long to retrain your taste buds.

● Herbalism can be very helpful, but it is important to consult a herbalist for individually tailored advice. Garlic, for example, has a proven ability to lower a raised blood pressure. Lime flower blossoms may be recommended where high blood pressure is linked with anxiety and stress but drink no more than three cups of infusion or herb tea daily except under the advice of a qualified herbalist.

● Take regular, gentle exercise.

● Aromatherapy: rosewood has been shown to be effective in lowering high blood pressure during pregnancy. Use under the supervision of a qualified aromatherapist. Care needs to be taken if you are also taking drugs to lower blood pressure. Other aromatherapy essential oils that can help after the 16th week of pregnancy include geranium, lavender and lemon.

● Floatation therapy can significantly lower high blood pressure and also helps you to relax.

● Meditation and visualisation are helpful and can be combined with floatation therapy.

● Yoga is excellent for relieving stress and reducing high blood pressure.

● The Alexander technique can help to relieve high blood pressure.

● Blue or indigo can be used in colour therapy to lower a high blood pressure.

- Other complementary therapies that can help include cymatics, healing, qigong, reflexology and reiki.

GESTATIONAL DIABETES

Gestational diabetes is a form of sugar diabetes (diabetes mellitus) that comes on during pregnancy. It affects around 5 per cent of previously non-diabetic women and occurs when the pancreas gland does not make enough insulin hormone to cope with the extra demands of pregnancy. Insulin is needed for cells to absorb glucose from the circulation, and during diabetes the blood glucose levels rise whilst cell glucose levels fall. Cell metabolism then becomes abnormal as a result of not getting enough fuel.

Gestational diabetes tends to appear during the second half of pregnancy and is more common in women who:

- are over the age of 25 years;
- have a family history of diabetes;
- are overweight or who put on a lot of weight during pregnancy;
- are carrying a large baby.

Women with gestational diabetes are able to have a successful pregnancy as long as their blood sugar levels are well controlled. If blood sugar levels are allowed to remain high, however, the baby may absorb excess glucose when its own pancreas starts making insulin. This can lead to an unusually large baby. Alternatively, the placenta may not work properly so the baby is unusually small.

Gestational diabetes is linked with an increased risk of:
- infections (e.g. cystitis and thrush);
- excessive production of amniotic fluid (polyhydramnios);
- pre-eclampsia (a serious disease of pregnancy, in which

there is high blood pressure, fluid retention and protein in the urine);

- eclampsia (an advanced form of pre-eclampsia in which fits occur);
- a build-up of acid and poisons in the body (ketoacidosis);
- kidney problems;
- miscarriage;
- preterm labour;
- a difficult labour;
- instrumental delivery (forceps or caesarean section);
- stillbirth;
- a baby with congenital abnormalities.

Most problems are successfully avoided by keeping blood sugar levels within the normal range and attending for all necessary antenatal check-ups. It is therefore vital to follow any advice and treatment recommended by your doctor or obstetrician. Most women with gestational diabetes have a mild form that can be controlled by careful diet. A dietician will advise you on how to eat healthily. Sometimes, however, regular insulin injections are needed.

Approximately 1–2 per cent of women who become pregnant are already known to have diabetes. Many hospitals offer preconceptual care clinics especially for diabetic patients. Ideally, diabetic women should carefully plan their pregnancies so they occur when their glucose control is stable. This can be monitored by assessing blood levels of a substance (glycosylated haemoglobin) that indicates how good your sugar control has been in recent weeks. Throughout your pregnancy, you will usually be cared for by both an obstetrician and a physician specialising in diabetes. It is vital that your blood glucose levels are tightly controlled.

In true gestational diabetes, blood sugar levels return to normal soon after delivery. Occasionally blood sugar levels remain high and continued diabetic treatment is needed. Gestational diabetes is a sign that your pancreas cannot cope with extra strain, and three out of four women who developed it go on to have mature onset diabetes in later life. This is usually controlled by diet and tablets alone.

- Stevia is an exciting plant from the rainforests of Paraguay and Southern Brazil. Its leaves contain a substance known as stevioside that is at least 100 times sweeter than cane sugar. These naturally sweet leaves can be used as a calorie-free sugar substitute that does not leave an aftertaste like most artificial sweeteners. Stevia also has other health benefits as it has recently been shown to protect against tooth decay. It is safe for use during pregnancy, and by diabetics. In Paraguay, Stevia is actually prescribed for diabetics as it is believed to normalise high blood sugar levels in its own right. Sugar provides 200–300 kcal per day in the average diet. This can be significantly reduced by for example, adding one or two dried leaves to your teapot during brewing, using powdered leaves when cooking, or adding a pinhead sized amount of Stevia extract to sweeten a cup of tea or coffee. Stevia is available as dried leaves (containing 10 per cent stevioside), powdered extract or liquid extract (dark or clear). Available by mail order from Rio Trading, Tel: (01273) 570987.
- Cymatics, crystal therapy, floatation therapy, healing, reflexology and reiki may be of benefit.

THRUSH

Vaginal thrush is due to infection with a yeast-like fungus, *Candida albicans*, which thrives in warm, moist places. It lives happily in or on the body of most of the population, usually without causing harm. When it overgrows, however, it can produce vaginal soreness, itching and a discharge like cottage cheese. Thrush is especially common during pregnancy, when hormonal changes mean the sugar content of vaginal cells is higher than normal. Recurrent thrush may be linked with lack of iron needed by white blood cells to help fight fungal infections.

- Increase your intake of dietary iron (e.g. seafood, red meat, poultry, nuts, wholegrains and green leafy vegetables), and vitamin C (e.g. citrus fruit, berry fruits and kiwi fruit), which boosts absorption of iron from the gut.
- A good vitamin and mineral supplement designed for pregnancy that includes iron is also a good idea.
- Avoid tight underwear, especially nylon pantyhose or tight trousers.
- Avoid getting hot and sweaty—use panty-liners and change them frequently.
- Boil your cotton underwear or hot-iron the gussets, as modern low temperature (40 °C/104° F) washing machine cycles do not kill *Candida* spores and recurrent thrush may be due to reinfection from your underclothes.
- Although there is no scientific evidence to support dietary changes, some women have found it helpful to follow a yeast-free diet. Others avoid alcohol, mushrooms, sugary foods, tea, coffee and chocolate. Eat a wholefood diet of saladstuff, fruit, vegetables, pulses and wholegrain cereals instead.
- Avoid sugar in your diet—use the natural sweetener Stevia instead (see p. 189).
- Try to avoid stress—make time for regular exercise, rest and relaxation.
- Avoid bath additives and vaginal deodorants, which upset your natural acid and bacterial balance.
- Ask your partner to use an antifungal cream as men can harbour yeasts without developing symptoms, so they keep passing spores back when making love.
- Aromatherapy: after the first 16 weeks of pregnancy, you

can add two drops each of bergamot, lavender and ger-anium essential oils to 30 ml carrier oil and add this to your bath water. Lie in the water and soak for 20 minutes. You can also add two drops of any of these antifungal oils to a little vitamin E cream, live 'bio' yoghurt or KY (or a similar) jelly and apply to the vulval area. Use as often as necessary to help relieve symptoms, especially itching.

- Homoeopathy (take six times a day for up to five days), as follows:
  — for vaginal candida with a milky, itchy discharge, especially if linked with premenstrual headache, stress, overwork or pregnancy, take Calcarea car-bonica;
  — for vaginal candida with an offensive discharge that is worse after making love take Sepia;
  — for vaginal candida with burning pains, especially if linked with stress or another illness (e.g. for which antibiotics were taken), take Sulphur;
  — for a copious, irritant, itchy discharge take Helonias;
  — for candida unresponsive to treatment take Candida albicans.
- Naturopathy: many cases of vaginal thrush are linked with low levels of friendly bacteria (*Lactobacillus acidophilus*) in the vagina and bowel. Eating live 'bio' yoghurt daily can help to restore bacterial balance and reduce the likeli-hood of recurrent thrush symptoms. In addition, you may also benefit from a yoghurt-like liquid supplement (Yakult) containing a culture of *Lactobacillus casei* Shirota. Sup-plements are also available in health food shops containing *Lactobacillus acidophilus*, *Lactobacillus bulgaricus* and related species such as *Bifidobacterium bifidum* and *Bifid-obacterium longum*. These can be taken in powder or cap-sule form, or used to make your own yoghurt cultures. Probiotic fruit juices fortified with *Lactobacilli* are also available in some areas (ProViva).

- Crystal therapy: carry a carnelian with you at all times.
- Other complementary therapies that can help include cymatics, healing, reiki and reflexology.

PREGNANCY-ASSOCIATED OSTEOPOROSIS

Osteoporosis during pregnancy is increasingly common. A developing baby has a high calcium requirement as the bones develop. If calcium is lacking from the diet, it will be leached from the mother's own bones and teeth—one reason why visits to the dentist are free during pregnancy and for a year afterwards. This mineral drain is significant and can weaken the bones enough to cause fractures; hundreds of cases are thought to occur every year during the last three months of pregnancy or in the early breast-feeding period. Unfortunately, symptoms are often misdiagnosed as pregnancy-associated back pain or even as postnatal depression. In one case, a new mother's bone mass was found to have thinned to 50 per cent of the normal value for her age after delivery of her child.

Most women recover any lost bone mass spontaneously after childbirth so long as they have a high calcium intake and regular exercise. Human breast milk contains 25–35 mg calcium per 100 ml (150–210 mg per pint) and affected mothers are strongly advised not to breast feed, as this is a further drain on calcium stores. For women who do not develop pregnancy-associated osteoporosis, however, new research suggests that bone loss during extended periods of breast feeding and closely spaced pregnancies is unlikely to have a lasting effect on the bones as long as they follow a healthy, calcium-rich diet. The best way to ensure a good calcium intake during pregnancy is to drink an extra pint of skimmed or semi-skimmed milk per day.

For more information see *The Osteoporosis Prevention Guide* by Dr Sarah Brewer (London: Souvenir Press).

- Consult a naturopath for full dietary and lifestyle advice.
- Other complementary therapies that can help include cymatics, healing, reiki, reflexology and t'ai chi.

BACK PAIN

Back pain affects most women towards the end of pregnancy as their posture changes—especially if they were unfit before pregnancy. Factors contributing to back pain include poor muscle tone, softening ligaments as delivery approaches, and the postural changes needed to compensate for your changing centre of gravity as baby and womb enlarge.

- Make sure you sleep on a good quality mattress such as one made of heat- and pressure-sensitive viscoelastic polymers (see p. 178).
- Eat more oily fish (e.g. salmon, mackerel, herrings and sardines), which contain building blocks for hormone-like substances (prostaglandins) that help to damp down joint inflammation and pain.
- Improve your posture by keeping your spine straight when walking and avoid slouching your shoulders.
- Wear flat or low shoes.
- Lift loads correctly: bend at the knees and hips, keep your back straight and upright and slowly straighten your legs as you rise.
- When sitting, keep square on the chair with your bottom well back and your spine upright. Use the chair arms to take some of the weight off your shoulders and lower back.
- Glucosamine is a natural substance formed from a sugar and an amino acid that is needed in the body to produce molecules (glycosaminoglycans) essential for healing damaged joints. Although your body can make glucosamine itself from a sugar (glucose) and an amino acid (glutamine), this is a slow process and glucosamine is often in

short supply. Glucosamine supplements improve the quality and thickness of cartilage and synovial fluid (the 'joint oil') so it is more protective. They also strengthen the jelly-like centre of intervertebral discs in danger of prolapse. Furthermore, supplements can boost joint healing—and are often more effective than painkillers. Eight out of ten users notice a significant improvement within two weeks.

- Acupuncture can ease back pain and is especially useful where tissues are so painful that back massage or manipulation cannot be carried out initially.
- The Alexander technique aims to improve poor posture and faulty body movements. By teaching you to stand and move correctly it can help a wide variety of conditions, including recurrent back pain and joint problems.
- Some essential oils are excellent at warming tissues and relieving back pain—in fact, many form the basis of traditional medical liniments. Essential oils that can be used to treat back pain after the 16th week of pregnancy include ginger, lavender, chamomile or rosemary (see p. 72).
- Floatation therapy allows you to lie on your back in a natural, comfortable, supported position that can help to relieve back pain.
- Homoeopathy: take 6c strength three times daily for up to five days, as follows:
  - for lower back pain that radiates to both hips take Kali carbonicum;
  - for low back pain relieved by firm pressure take Natrum muriaticum;
  - for backache worse on starting to move take Rhus toxicodendron.
- If you are planning to hire a transcutaneous electrical nerve stimulation (TENS) machine for pain relief during delivery, you may find it helpful to use it earlier in pregnancy to relieve your back ache, too.

- Crystal therapy: carry a ruby or garnet with you at all times.
- Other complementary therapies that can help established back pain include chiropractic, osteopathy, cranial osteopathy, craniosacral therapy, cymatics, healing, hellerwork, massage, reiki and reflexology.

SYMPHYSIS PUBIS PAIN

Towards the end of pregnancy a natural hormone, relaxin, is secreted that softens ligaments so the pelvic bones can move apart more easily during childbirth. The pubic joint at the front of the pelvis (symphysis pelvis) is especially affected and this can cause pain in the pubic area, which is worse on walking or moving the legs. Pain may also be felt in the lower back, groin and inner thighs.

- Take plenty of rest and avoid lifting, standing and walking as much as possible.
- Homoeopathy: take the following:
    - Hypericum 30c two or three times a day;
    - Arnica 30c two or three times a day.
- Crystal therapy: carry a ruby or garnet with you at all times.
- Other therapies that can help include acupuncture, the Alexander technique, massage, osteopathy, chiropractic, craniosacral therapy, hellerwork, healing, reiki and reflexology.

When pain is troublesome, ask your doctor or midwife to refer you for physiotherapy, as being fitted with a support belt will help.

FOOD CRAVINGS

Food cravings can occur during pregnancy for foods such as sardines, oranges, ice-cream, and cheese and pickle sandwiches. These are not uncommon, and in most cases little harm comes from indulging them within moderation. Pica is a form of food craving that can occur during pregnancy in which there is a strong urge to eat non-food substances such as clay, chalk, earth or coal. Pica is sometimes a symptom of iron deficiency and if it occurs iron supplements are recommended. Try to resist the urge to eat non-food substances as they may cause harm to the developing baby.

- Specific homoeopathic remedies can help to reduce cravings for foods and for non-foods (see p. 119).
- Consult a naturopath for individual dietary and lifestyle advice.
- Other complementary therapies that can help include cymatics, healing, reiki and reflexology.

SWOLLEN ANKLES

Swollen ankles may develop towards the end of pregnancy when the enlarged uterus compresses veins draining fluid back from the legs. If swelling persists, and if puffy fingers occur as well, it is important to have your blood pressure checked by your doctor or midwife to rule out pre-eclampsia.

- Take regular, gentle exercise.
- Rest with your feet up for at least half an hour, twice a day.
- Acupuncture can be highly effective.
- Aromatherapy: geranium and rosemary are good for fluid retention during pregnancy. **NB: Rosemary is not to be used if the woman has any degree of hypertension.**
- Herbalism: Cornsilk and fennel have mild diuretic proper-

ties. An infusion of cornsilk in water can help mild fluid retention during pregnancy. Drink no more than four cups of cornsilk infusion daily during pregnancy except under the advice of a qualified herbalist.

- Other complementary therapies that may help include: cymatics, homoeopathy, healing, hellerwork, reiki, reflexology, massage, ta'i chi and yoga.

ASTHMA

Asthma is a long-term, inflammatory disease of the lungs. The exact cause is unknown, but the inflammation is thought to be linked to an overactive immune system. The lining of the airways becomes red and swollen and produces increased amounts of mucus. Once irritation sets in, the airways become increasingly sensitive to a wide range of triggers such as exercise, emotion and exposure to the cold. If left untreated, asthma causes recurrent attacks of breathlessness, wheezing or coughing. Asthma is especially common in women—two out of three sufferers are female. During pregnancy, a woman's asthma may worsen, improve or stay the same but usually returns to normal within three months of giving birth. Half of women with asthma find each pregnancy affects their asthma in the same way, but the other half find their symptoms differ from pregnancy to pregnancy.

A recent study involving 28 women with moderate to severe asthma found they were more likely to develop worsening asthma symptoms when pregnant with a girl than with a boy. This effect did not have a psychological basis as none of the women questioned knew the sex of her baby before delivery. The researchers suggest that subtle changes in hormone levels may be involved. Most of the women taking part in the study answered questions about their asthma between weeks 12 and 16 of pregnancy. This is a time when male babies produce a natural surge of male hormones known as androgens. It is possible that these hormone changes affect the mother's symptoms in some way and further investigation is needed.

Common triggers for asthma include:

Allergic asthma
- grass and tree pollen;
- house dust mite;
- animal fur;
- fungal spores and moulds;
- certain foods;
- work hazards e.g. some chemicals.

Non-allergic asthma
- viral infections e.g. colds;
- cigarette smoke;
- cold or damp air;
- exercise;
- strong emotions e.g. laughter;
- cosmetics and perfumes;
- air pollution;
- hormonal changes e.g. periods or pregnancy in women;
- acid reflux (indigestion);
- some drugs;
- stress.

To help reduce asthma symptoms:

- Avoid factors that trigger your asthma.
- Try to avoid exposure to cigarette smoke and traffic fumes.
- Keep the home as dust free as possible. Dusting with a damp cloth and using a vacuum cleaner with a special filter will help.
- Put special covers over your mattress, pillow and duvet to overcome bed mites.

- Wash the family cat or dog at least once a week (ask a family member to do this when you are not around).
- Breathing exercises may help you relax and control your breathing better.
- Fish oils contain anti-inflammatory substances and seem to protect against asthma—try eating more oily fish.
- A diet rich in vitamins C and E seems to protect against asthma.
- Homoeopathy may help patients with allergic asthma, when used together with standard treatments. Consult a homoeopathic practitioner for advice.
- Always take prescribed medications exactly as your doctor advises.
- Complementary therapies that can help include acupuncture, aromatherapy, cymatics, qigong, healing, reiki and reflexology.

RHINITIS

Some women suffer nasal congestion (rhinitis) during pregnancy with difficulty in breathing that may interfere with sleep. Symptoms are due to increased blood flow during pregnancy, which makes the lining of the nose swell. In severe cases, the blocked nasal passages may reduce drainage from the sinuses so that sinusitis results.

- Steam inhalations help by moistening and thinning secretions to get them moving.
- Try using a humidifier or a negative ioniser in your bedroom.
- Aromatherapy: place one drop each of lemon, lavender and tea tree oil on a tissue (or in hot water) and inhale.
- Herbalism: lime flower blossoms reduce nasal secretions and are also helpful for cold symptoms. Drink no more

than three cups of infusion or herb tea daily except under the advice of a qualified herbalist.

- Other complementary therapies that can help include acupuncture, acupressure, chiropractic, healing, homoeopathy, osteopathy, cranial osteopathy, craniosacral therapy, reiki and reflexology.

BREECH BABY

A breech baby is one who fails to turn properly so that the bottom, rather than the baby's head, presents downwards. A breech position occurs in 3 to 4 per cent of pregnancies. In around 60 per cent of pregnancies, a baby will turn by itself after 32 weeks. A further 25 per cent will turn after 36 weeks.

- Walk regularly each day to help encourage your baby to turn.
- Acupuncturists have had great success in using moxibustion to help turn a breech baby (see p. 65).
- Homoeopathy: take Caulophyllum (blue cohosh) at the 30c potency twice a week. After turning, Pulsatilla 6c may be taken twice a day to help encourage the baby to maintain the right position.
- Other complementary therapies that can help include hellerwork, reflexology and reiki.

CHAPTER 6

Natural Approaches to Childbirth

Childbirth can be an exciting, frightening, exhilarating and fulfilling experience—all at the same time. Thanks to changing policies, women now have more control over the process, which reduces the fear and increases the fulfilment. You will be encouraged to draw up a birth plan that states how—in an ideal world—you would like your labour to proceed. This can include having an alternative practitioner with you during your confinement, and the positions you wish to adopt for labour and delivery. If you wish to have a therapist with you during labour in a hospital unit, you will usually need to arrange this beforehand and obtain permission as sometimes there is a limit on the number of people allowed in the room with you. The National Childbirth Trust provides a leaflet, 'Making a Birth Plan', sponsored by Tesco supermarkets, which suggests that a birth plan should be written at about 36 weeks of pregnancy, although it is often helpful to start thinking about it and discussing it from 28 weeks onwards. It is important to remain flexible in your wishes, however. Different women have different needs during pregnancy and it is not always possible to tell what these will be in advance. Even the best-laid plans may have to be abandoned if you are faced with particular circumstances or complications at the time of delivery. If you have your heart set on a natural birth, but then need a forceps delivery or caesarean section, it is easy to feel you have somehow failed when, of course, you haven't, as you will have succeeded in bringing a wonderful new life into the world. Holistic therapies help to put these aspects of childbirth into perspective yet at the same time help you to relax so that complications are less likely to mean a deviation from your birth plan.

ACTIVE BIRTH

The active birth movement was founded in the late 1970s by Janet Balaskas, who encouraged women to use more natural upright positions and to remain mobile during labour so gravity assists the process. Active birth classes are widely available; they prepare you physically and emotionally for birth, as well as providing support during pregnancy through weekly classes of easy and relaxing 'gravitational' yoga, which is ideally suited for pregnancy. According to Janet, 'These yoga-based exercises help to relieve tightness and tension in the body, improve flexibility, encourage good breathing and circulation. You will learn to be comfortable in upright positions and to manage pain in labour with breathing and relaxation.' Active birth classes have an open-minded approach, covering the same ground as traditional antenatal classes, with an additional emphasis on upright labour and birth positions, relaxation, breathing and the use of warm water during labour (they offer a water birth pool hire service). It's best to join active birth classes as early as possible in pregnancy, although it is never too late to join. For further information, contact the Active Birth Centre (see Useful addresses, p. 221).

STAGES OF LABOUR

There are three mains stages to childbirth:

Stage 1: Your waters break and regular contractions start to push your baby down against the cervix, which slowly widens to a diameter of around 10 cm (4 in).

202

Stage 2: Your womb continues to contract and your baby passes down the birth canal to be born—usually head first. The umbilical cord is then cut.

Stage 3: The placenta (afterbirth) is delivered.

There are two methods of delivering the placenta. In the 'managed' third stage, a drug (Syntometrine) is injected into your thigh as soon as your baby's shoulders are born. This helps your uterus to contract strongly and both reduces the risk of haemorrhage and eases expulsion of the placenta. After delivery, the umbilical cord is cut and the midwife delivers the placenta around five minutes later by gentle traction. In a 'natural' third stage of labour, the umbilical cord is not cut after birth. Instead, the baby is put to the breast and is encouraged to suckle. Breast feeding stimulates secretion of a hormone (oxytocin), which causes the womb to contract. The midwife then waits until the placenta naturally separates from the uterus, which may be 10 to 90 minutes later. The way this third stage of delivery is managed is one of the things you may wish to discuss with your midwife and include in your birth plan. However, you can have a natural third stage only if you have had a natural labour, without drugs or an epidural.

NATURAL PAIN RELIEF

A surprisingly wide range of complementary therapies offer natural means of relieving the pain of labour. These include:

- relaxation and breathing techniques (e.g. autogenic training and floatation);
- acupuncture;
- Alexander technique;
- aromatherapy;
- autogenic training;

- herbalism;
- homoeopathy;
- hypnotherapy;
- massage;
- meditation;
- reflexology.

Consult a qualified therapist to see what individual help can be offered to you while preparing for labour, and during childbirth.

In addition, a water birth and TENS are worth considering.

THE ROLE OF DIFFERENT THERAPIES IN THE BIRTH PROCESS

Acupuncture

In preparing for childbirth, therapist Keith Wright feels it is important to open up your heart–uterus connection (see p. 46) and to initiate your nesting instinct during the last six or eight weeks of pregnancy. Acupuncture can encourage the baby's head to engage and can be used to induce labour at nature's pace, as an alternative to a hospital induction. Some midwives will use this for women who are 'post-term'.

During the first stage of labour, acupuncture helps to relax and soften the cervix to aid dilation. Both acupuncture and electroacupuncture can be used to increase uterine contractions and have also been found effective in clinical trials for relieving back pain and the pain of contractions. Electroacupuncture is particularly helpful, but is not ideal in labour because of the need to be attached to wires and the unpredictable pain relief achieved. As well as helping to calm the mother and baby during labour, acupuncture can reinforce maternal energy levels to help prevent a prolonged labour.

During the first stage of labour, acupuncture can strengthen weak uterine contractions to increase their efficiency and can speed delivery, as well as relieving palpitations, breathlessness, upper abdominal pain or excessive bleeding.

During the third stage of labour, acupuncture can induce placental separation, relieve after-pains and stem haemorrhaging.

Alexander technique
The Alexander technique encourages pelvic floor exercises in preparation for childbirth, and—like the active birth movement—recommends that women stay upright during labour so gravity can naturally assist the birthing process.

Aromatherapy
The Pregnancy Shop (see p. 220) supplies Labour Massage Oil combining rose (to prepare the uterus for labour), petitgrain and lavandin. During labour, you can use a massage oil made from lavender 12 drops, clary sage 12 drops and jasmine rose four drops in 100 ml of carrier oil to help strengthen uterine contractions and give a feeling of well-being.

Frankincense, one drop in the palm of the hand or on a tissue, is helpful for calming and hyperventilation.

Nutmeg, two drops applied over the suprapubic and sacral regions as a compress, is helpful as an analgesic but should not be used if you have received a pethidine injection, or are likely to do so.

Bach flower essences
The Bach flower essence Mimulus will help you overcome any fears about giving birth or about the effect that pregnancy is having on you. Mimulus is the remedy for 'known' fears—in other words, fears that have a definite cause you can name. Red Chestnut may also be used to ease any exaggerated fears for the welfare of the baby. This is another fear remedy, like Mimulus, but is specifically for people who are anxious not about their own welfare but about the well-being of someone

else. If you are anxious about your own *and* your baby's health, then Red Chestnut and Mimulus together may be recommended.

Cymatics
Cymatics can be used to help provide pain relief during labour.

Hellerwork
Hellerwork can be helpful for encouraging a baby's head to engage in preparation for childbirth.

Herbalism
Raspberry leaf taken in the form of tea or tablets helps to soften the neck of the womb in preparation for delivery. It should be taken daily during the last eight weeks of pregnancy. It should not be taken during early pregnancy. It seems to reduce the duration and pain of childbirth. Mothers who have taken it often say their contractions were relatively pain free and their baby was born within just a few hours of labour starting. It is thought to work by strengthening the longitudinal muscles of the uterus to increase the force of uterine contractions.

Homoeopathy
For painful Braxton–Hicks contractions of the uterus towards the end of pregnancy, the homoeopathic remedy Cimicifuga can help. Arnica 6c taken twice a day in the last month will tone the uterus, and prepare the muscles for the birth. According to homoeopath Tricia Longworth, because Arnica is so effective for shock and bruising, it prepares the baby's head for the journey through the birth canal and minimises the effect of birth trauma so the baby can settle more easily into its new world. For the mother, Arnica helps prevent uterine haemorrhage as the placenta sheds away from the lining of the womb.

Dr Peter Webb recommends Caulophyllum (blue cohosh)

in preparation for labour. Start taking it from the 37th week of pregnancy, at the 30c potency twice a week (but not on consecutive days) until labour starts. This makes for an easier labour by strengthening uterine muscular activity and softening the neck of the womb. It helps the baby to descend more quickly, reducing the need for episiotomy, forceps and caesarean section. Caulophyllum can also be used where labour is delayed and for after pains.

During labour itself, remedies are available to help deal with complications such as retained placenta, ineffectual contractions, prolonged labour or haemorrhage, but these need to be prescribed by an experienced homoeopath.

Dr Peter Webb recommends taking Arnica 30c and Hypericum 30c as soon as labour becomes established. Arnica can be taken every hour during the birth, and three times a day for a few days after the labour. Arnica reduces blood loss and bruising, and will also stop a precipitate labour. The Hypericum will help heal any vulval damage, reduce sacral pain and will help skin healing if an episiotomy or caesarean section are necessary.

Belladonna can provide pain relief during labour if associated with a red face, moaning and irrational behaviour.

Staphysagria 30c should be taken on the fourth day after delivery to prevent the baby blues. It will also help heal the urethra should catheterisation have taken place during delivery.

If you have an episiotomy, or tear, try bathing the wound with a few drops of Hypercal (Hypericum and Calendula officinalis) tincture in warm water to hasten healing.

Hypnotherapy
Hypnotherapy and self-hypnosis can help to prepare you for childbirth, encourage relaxation and reduce pain perception.

Massage

Massage is relaxing and stimulates release of the body's natural painkillers to relieve discomfort during the end of pregnancy, and lift a depressed mood. It also helps to develop muscles and can help to prepare a woman for childbirth, especially one who leads a sedentary life and has not exercised much during her pregnancy. The London College of Massage recommends massaging oil into the perineum (area between the vagina and rectum) daily for six weeks before term to help soften and elasticise the tissues so that tearing and episiotomy are less likely. Use lavender and geranium essential oils diluted with wheatgerm oil, and massage daily for five to ten minutes starting six weeks before your baby is due (see p. 133 for full instructions).

According to the Massage Therapy Institute of Great Britain, massage during labour helps to relieve pain by stimulating production of endorphins—the body's own pain-relieving chemicals. As a result, massage can reduce the need for pain relief during labour. During the first stage of labour, massaging the shoulders and upper and lower spine can help relaxation, while massage that starts at the top of the body and moves down to the feet can help to release energy and accelerate labour. Pressing deeply with the thumbs into the centre of each buttock can help to relieve lower back pain, as can applying a deep, firm pressure on the sacrum with the heel of one hand. In the second stage, massaging the inside of the thighs will help, while massaging almond oil into the perineum helps it to stretch and become more elastic. This can reduce the need for an episiotomy.

Qigong

Qigong uses meditation and posture to help you to relax, to improve posture, muscle control and breathing, and to breathe in a certain way. It helps to channel energy (*qi*), strengthen muscles, produce a feeling of lightness and calm the mind in preparation for labour.

Reflexology

Practitioners have found that stimulating the reflexology points linked with the pituitary gland in the brain can also stimulate the release of oxytocin to start contractions. Research also suggests that reflexology can stimulate weak uterine contractions and shorten the length of an average labour by as much as half, as well as reducing the need for pain relief. Many midwives also use reflexology to help with pain during labour.

Reiki

Reiki can help to reduce apprehension and fear during late pregnancy and prepare you for the impending labour through the deep relaxation, renewed balance and confidence reiki healing brings.

TENS

TENS is a drug-free way to relieve back pain that is well accepted by the medical profession. Four pads are placed on your back (or over painful areas) and a small electric current pulses through these to stimulate nerve endings in the skin. This sends pain-blocking signals to the brain and temporarily numbs surrounding tissues. TENS is used to relieve any musculoskeletal pain (e.g. general back pain, sports injuries, sciatica, arthritis or tennis elbow) and is also used during childbirth. TENS machines are widely available for sale or hire.

WATER LABOUR

Being suspended in warm water during labour can ease the pain of contractions and help you to stay comfortable. Just having a warm bath will help, but many hospital units have their own water pool in which you can undergo labour, assuming it is not being used when you need it. You can also arrange to hire a water pool in advance to ensure that one is available for you (e.g. through the Active Birth Centre; see p. 221). Your midwife will be able to tell you about local facilities. Some women choose to have the delivery itself in a water pool. You will need to be supervised by a midwife experienced in water births and to have a full discussion beforehand about the benefits versus the risks before deciding whether or not to do this.

CHAPTER 7

After Your Baby is Born

After your baby is born, complementary therapies can help you return to normal, help with breast feeding and reduce the risk of the baby blues and postnatal depression.

THE BENEFITS OF DIFFERENT THERAPIES

Acupuncture
Acupuncture is helpful after childbirth in relieving postnatal depression, insomnia, urinary and bowel problems as well as helping your return to a normal non-pregnant balance of health. If you have had a caesarean section, acupuncture can hasten healing.

Aromatherapy
After childbirth, an aromatherapy bath containing diluted lavender, geranium and rose essential oils will help you re-establish your normal non-pregnant balance.

Diluted lavender oil is recommended for perineal care, while orange, mandarin, neroli, bergamot, geranium, rose, jasmine, sandalwood or ylang-ylang are useful for keeping depression at bay.

Bach flower remedies
The Bach flower essence Olive is helpful for mental and physical tiredness following delivery. Unaccountable depression can be helped with Mustard, difficulties adjusting

eased with Walnut, and irritability washed away with Impatiens or Beech.

Cranial osteopathy

Cranial osteopathy can help you overcome childbirth and may also be used on infants to correct distortions caused by a prolonged or difficult birth, and to relieve the irritability and colic that may result.

Massage

During the first few weeks after childbirth, a daily shoulder, neck and back massage will help you sleep, renew your energy levels and improve your physical and mental health.

Many other therapies are also helpful immediately after childbirth, including chiropractic, osteopathy, craniosacral therapy, reflexology and reiki.

BREAST FEEDING

The ideal way to feed your baby is as nature intended, with breast milk. Breast milk is the most nutritionally complete food you can offer your infant for both physical and mental development. It contains:

- all the energy, protein, fat, sugar, vitamins, minerals and fluids your baby needs for the first six months;
- antibodies to protect against disease;
- active scavenger immune cells to protect against disease;
- natural antibacterial and antiviral substances;
- essential fatty acids that are vital for your baby's brain development;
- growth factors that influence growth and maturation of your baby.

The ideal way to breast feed is to supply your baby with milk whenever needed, which is known as 'on demand'. New government guidelines recommend putting your baby to the breast within an hour of birth. Ideally, your baby should be breast fed exclusively for four to six months. Breast milk should then continue to be given after weaning on to solids, up until at least your child's first birthday. Many children continue to enjoy the benefits of breast feeding until the age of two years or beyond.

Every woman who is planning to have a baby should read *Breast is Best* by Drs Penny and Andrew Stanway (London: Pan) for a complete picture of breast feeding, including why it is by far the healthiest option for both mother and baby, hints and tips on how to get started, how to do it successfully—including when working—and how to overcome problems.

Diet

While pregnant and breast feeding, consider taking essential fatty acid supplements containing long-chain fatty acids (e.g. Efanatal, Milkarra in the UK; Neuromins in the US) designed to enhance the amount of essential fatty acids—essential for brain development—your baby receives.

Herbalism

Drinking fennel or dill tea after delivery helps to stimulate the production of breast milk. Drink no more than two cups of fennel tea daily during pregnancy except under the advice of a qualified herbalist. Agnus castus both stimulates milk production and can boost a low sex drive postnatally.

OVERCOMING BREAST PROBLEMS

Inflammation of the breast—mastitis—can occur at any time when breast feeding. In half of cases, the problem is due to engorgement or a blocked duct, while in the other half it is due to infection.

Engorgement

Engorged breasts can occur at any time if milk is allowed to build up. This can cause:

- hot, swollen, painful breasts with red, shiny skin;
- dilated reservoirs and ducts feeling like hard lumps or cords under the skin;
- feelings of being hot, sweaty and shivery;
- thirst, which you should quench by drinking as much as you need.

Unlike a blocked duct and infection, engorgement usually affects both breasts. If the pressure isn't relieved, your milk supply may dry up. If you want to continue breast feeding, feed your baby frequently, whenever your breasts feel full—even if you have to wake your baby to do so. As engorgement tends to flatten the nipples, expressing a little milk first, by hand, will help baby get a good latch. Alternatively, express excess milk with a pump. Empty your breasts enough for any lumps to disappear. Reduce discomfort by cooling your breasts with a flannel soaked in ice-cold water, or by using an 'ice pack' (e.g. a bag of frozen peas wrapped in a tea towel).

Homoeopathy

Hypercal (Hypericum and Calendula officinalis) tincture in warm water is good for both sore nipples and nappy rash.

Aromatherapy

Benzoin four drops, rose three drops and Roman chamomile two drops applied in a cream or lotion can ease sore nipples and breasts. The cream or lotion must be removed completely before breast feeding.

Blocked duct

A blocked duct can be due to pressure from a poorly fitting bra or from incomplete draining of a duct after engorgement. It usually affects only one breast and causes localised mastitis with:

- a small area of redness, tenderness and lumpiness;
- increasing pain as milk is let down when feeding;
- flu-like symptoms.

If left untreated, a blocked duct can lead to more severe inflammation, and even a fever, owing to leakage of trapped milk into breast tissues. Stagnant milk can also become infected. Feed your baby at the affected breast as often as you can, offering this breast first. During the feed, gently but firmly massage the lump towards the nipple with your fingers. Vary your position with each feed (e.g. tuck baby under one arm, lie on your side, or even kneel over baby so your breast is directly overhead) to alter the way the ducts are drained. After finishing a feed, express any remaining milk with a pump. Check your bra is properly fitted and that there are no tight bands across the top. Relieve discomfort by immersing breasts in comfortably hot water (e.g. a bath), or wash with a flannel soaked in hot water. If the problem doesn't settle within 24 hours, seek medical advice as you may need antibiotics.

Mastitis with infection

Mastitis due to infection usually only affects one breast. Symptoms can include:

- a hot, swollen, painful breast with red, shiny skin;
- flu-like symptoms with shivering, aching and a fever;
- nausea and sometimes vomiting;
- sometimes being able to squeeze pus from the nipple.

If only a small area of one breast is infected, it may resemble a blocked duct. If the whole breast is involved, it may resemble

215

engorgement, although this usually only affects one side.

Acupuncture
Acupuncture can regulate the flow of breast milk and help to alleviate mastitis.

Aromatherapy
Roman chamomile three drops, peppermint two drops and geranium two drops applied as a compress can help.

SEEKING HELP

If symptoms do not improve quickly, or if they start to worsen, seek medical advice as antibiotics will be need to prevent abscess formation. If you are worried about painful breasts in any way, ask your doctor, midwife or health visitor for advice straight away. You can usually continue to feed your baby when you have infected mastitis and are on antibiotics, but follow your doctor's advice—if bacterial counts are very high this may not be recommended.

Further Reading

Childbirth
BRADFORD, N., and CHAMBERLAIN, G. (1995). *Pain Relief in Childbirth*. London: HarperCollins.
BALASKAS, J. (1985). *Active Birth*. London: Thorsons.

COMPLEMENTARY THERAPIES

Alexander technique
MACHOVER, I., DRAKE, A., and DRAKE, J. (1993). *Pregnancy and Birth, the Alexander Way*. London: Robinson.

Aromatherapy
PRICE, S., and PRICE PARR, P. (1996). *Aromatherapy for Babies and Children*. London: Thorsons.
CLIFFORD, F. R. (1997). *Aromatherapy During your Pregnancy*. Saffron Walden: C. W. Daniel Co. Ltd.
FAWCETT, M. (1993). *Aromatherapy for Pregnancy and Childbirth*. Shaftesbury: Element.

Autogenic training
KANJI, N. (1997). Autogenic training. In *Journal of Complementary Therapies in Medicine*, **5**, 162–167.

Bach flower remedies
HOWARD, J. (1992). *Bach Flower Remedies for Women*. Saffron Walden: C. W. Daniel Co. Ltd.

217

BALL, S. (1999). *Principles of Bach Flower Therapy*. London: Thorsons.

BALL, S. (1998). *The Bach Remedies Workbook*. Saffron Walden: C. W. Daniel Co. Ltd.

HOWARD, J. (1994). *Growing up with Bach Flower Remedies*. Saffron Waldon: C. W. Daniel Co. Ltd.

Chiropractic

ANDREWS, E., and COURTENAY, A. (1999). *The Essentials of McTimoney Chiropractic—the Gentle Art of Whole Body Adjustment*. London: Thorsons.

Crystal therapy

MELODY. (1995). *Love is the Earth. A Kaleidoscope of Crystals Updated*. Colorado: Earth Love Publishing.

Hellerwork

GOLTEN, R. (1999). *The Owner's Guide to the Body*. London: Thorsons/HarperCollins.

Homoeopathy

WEBB, Dr P. (1999). *Homoeopathy for Midwives (and All Pregnant Women)*, 2nd edn. British Homoeopathic Association.

WEBB, Dr P. (1997). *The Family Encyclopedia of Homoeopathic Remedies*. London: Robinson.

ROSE, Dr B., and SCOTT-MONCRIEFF, Dr C. (1998). *Homoeopathy for Women*. London: Collins & Brown.

LOCKIE, Dr A., and GEDDES, Dr N. *The Women's Guide to Homeopathy*. London: Hamish Hamilton.

Kinesiology

For *Introduction to Kinesiology*, a 60-page booklet explaining the basics of AK and featuring the Emotional Stress Release technique, please send a cheque for £2.50 (inc. p&p) to

TASK Books 39 Browns Road, Surbiton, Surrey KT5 8ST. For *Your Breasts, What Every Women Needs to Know Now*, by Brian Butler, please send a cheque for £10 (inc. p&p) to TASK Books.

Massage
MAXWELL-HUDSON, C. (1988). *The Complete Book of Massage*. London: Dorling Kindersley.
MONTAGUE, Dr A. DO. *Touching, the Human Significance of the Skin*.

Prenatal stimulation
BREWER, Dr S. (1998). *Super Baby*. London: Thorsons.

Reflexology
HALL, N. *Reflexology for Women*. London: Thorsons.
Gateways to Health and Harmony with Reflexology. (available from the Holistic Healing Centre: 01279 429060)

Yoga
FREEDMAN, Dr F., and HALL, D. (1998). *Yoga for Pregnancy*. London: Ward Lock.
FREEDMAN, Dr. F., and HALL, D. *Postnatal Yoga*. London: Ward Lock.
BALASKAS, J. *Preparing for Birth with Yoga*. Shaftesbury: Element.
LINCOLN, F. *Easy Exercises for Pregnancy*. London: Frances Lincoln.

Useful Addresses

General

The Pregnancy Shop
Manor View, Claydon, Banbury, Oxfordshire OX17 1HH.
helpline: 0891-633473; orders and further information: 0870-1-668899
website: www.pregnancy.shop-com
The Pregnancy Shop is a unique mail order service that provides natural products to support women during their pregnancy and following the birth of their baby. All the products have been developed in co-operation with midwives, doctors and pregnant women. They include:

- the Feeling Lousy Kit—to relieve and revive during the early weeks of pregnancy;
- the Almost There Kit—to prepare a woman for and support her during labour;
- the New Arrival Kit—to relax, soothe and bond mother and baby;
- Inside Out Kit—containing PregVital vitamins, Milkarra (DHA oils) and Beautiful Belly Balm.

Some products are also sold individually, including:

- Get Better Down Under Gel;
- PregVital vitamins;

- Milkarra;
- BioZest Labour Drink;
- Acu-Magnets;
- Beautiful Belly Balm;
- Beautiful Baby Bottom Cream.

Active Birth Centre
25 Bickerton Road, London N19 4JT.
tel: 0171-561-9006; fax: 0171-561-9007
e-mail: mail@activebirthcentr.demon.co.uk
website: www.activebirthcentre.com
Helps prospective parents achieve an optimum pregnancy and labour by exploring alternatives and increasing awareness of the benefits of active birth and breast feeding. Provides information on active birth, yoga, baby massage and gymnastics plus a variety of alternative therapies, including homoeopathy and acupuncture, paediatric acupuncture and cranial osteopathy. Can provide water pools for birth.

Eating for Pregnancy Helpline: 0114-242-4084

Breast Feeding

Association of Breastfeeding Mothers (ABM)
PO Box 207, Bridgewater, TA6 7YT.
tel: 0171-813-1481
e-mail: abm@clara.net
website: hhtp;//home.clara.net/abm/
Promotes increased awareness of the benefits of breast feeding and how to do it. Runs a telephone counselling service.

La Leche League of Great Britain
Box BM 3424, London WC1N 3XX.
tel: 0171-242-1278
Provides information, support and personal help to women

who wish to breastfeed their babies through mother-to-mother support groups and a telephone helpline.

National Childbirth Trust (NCT)
Alexandra House, Oldham Terrace, London W3 6NH.
tel: 0181-992-2616; 0181-992-8637 (helpline
9.30 a.m.–4.30 p.m.); fax: 0181-992-5929
Offers information and support in pregnancy, childbirth and early parenthood, and to enable all parents to make informed choices. Provides antenatal classes, breast-feeding counselling, postnatal support and birth/parenthood education in schools. Provides a number of information leaflets, including 'Making a Birth Plan', 'Postnatal Depression', 'Breastfeeding: Returning to Work', 'Where shall I have my baby?' and 'Becoming a Dad'.

Acupuncture

Details of medically qualified acupuncturists can be obtained from:
The British Medical Acupuncture Society
Newton House, Newton Lane, Whitley, Warrington, Cheshire WA4 4JA.
tel: 01925-730727; fax: 01925-730492
e-mail: Bmasadmin@aol.com
URL: http://www.medicalacupuncture.co.uk
The British Medical Acupuncture Society (BMAS) represents medically qualified doctors who practise acupuncture alongside conventional medicine. The society was formed in 1980 with only a handful of members, since when its membership has grown to over 1600. The BMAS supports and encourages research into acupuncture so that we can all benefit from the most effective acupuncture treatments possible. Acupuncture is not considered appropriate for all conditions and practitioners are discouraged from making claims for the value of

acupuncture where there is no supporting evidence. The major-
ity of members are general practitioners, many of whom offer
acupuncture on the NHS. For details of medically qualified
acupuncturists in your area, contact the head office (details
elsewhere).

Dr Richard Halvorsen
The Holborn Medical Centre, 64 Lambs Conduit Street,
London WC1N 3LW.
tel: 0171-405-3541; fax: 0171-404-8198

Dr Richard Halvorsen is a GP practising in Central London.
After qualifying as a doctor in London in 1982, he studied
traditional Chinese acupuncture. More recently he has studied
different methods of acupuncture and has visited China to
learn how it is used there today. He is a member of the British
Medical Acupuncture Society and, like other members, advo-
cates the practice of evidence-based acupuncture. He offers
acupuncture to his NHS patients without charge, and privately
to others. He can be contacted at:

Zita West, 10 Harley Street, London W1.
Tel: 0171-467-8475.

Warwick Hospital: 01926-495321 ext. 4709

Details of qualified practitioners of traditional acupuncture can
be obtained from:
The British Acupuncture Council
Park House, 206–208 Latimer Road, London W10 6RE.
tel: 0181-964-0222; fax: 0181-964-0333
e-mail: info@acupuncture.org.uk
The British Acupuncture Council (BAcC) represents 1,800 acu-
puncturists *who have an extensive training in acupuncture and*
the western medical sciences appropriate to the practice of

acupuncture. Members practise a recognised and traditional style of diagnosis and treatment therapy. This type of therapy has been developed and refined over 2000 years in China and provides patients with an holistic approach to maintaining health and managing illness.

There is no government legislation in the UK covering acupuncture at present. This means that anyone, including doctors, physiotherapists etc. can give acupuncture treatment without any training whatsoever. The BAcC believes that anyone who wishes to provide acupuncture treatment should undertake an extensive training of at least two years full-time (or the part-time equivalent) irrespective *of any other medical training.*

The BAcC maintains standards of education, ethics, discipline and codes of practice to ensure the health and safety of the public at all times. It is also committed to promoting research and enhancing the role that traditional acupuncture can play in the health and well-being of the nation.

International College of Oriental Medicine
Green Hedges House, Green Hedges Lane, East Grinstead, West Sussex RH19 1DZ.
tel: 01342-313106
The College is a member of the British Acupuncture Council.

Keith Wright, MBAcA, lecturer at the ICOM, can be contacted at:

- Flint House, 41 High Street, Lewes, E. Sussex BN7 1UD (tel: 01273 473388)
- Gables Clinic, 108 High Street, Uckfield, E. Sussex TN22 1PX (tel: 01825 712895).
- Helios Clinic, 97 Camden Road, Tunbridge Wells, Kent TN1 2QR (tel: 01892 510950)

- The Acupuncture Clinic, 11 Normansland, Fairwarp TN22 3BS (tel: 01825 712895)

Contact the Association of Midwife Acupuncturists for details of midwives who offer acupuncture as part of their care. Contact: Sarah Budd on 01837-840424.

Three maternity units where acupuncture is offered on the NHS:
1 Derriford Hospital, Plymouth;
2 Warwick Maternity Hospital;
3 Obstetric Hospital, UCLH, London.

British Acupuncture Association and Register
34 Alderney Street, London, SW1V 4EU.
tel: 0171-834-1012
Information leaflets, booklets, register of qualified practitioners.
Tel: 01904-781630

Alexander Technique

The Society of Teachers of the Alexander Technique
20 London House, 266 Fulham Road, London SW10 9EL.
tel: 0171-351-0828

Aromatherapy

Aromatherapy Organisations Council
PO Box 19834, London SE25 6WF.
tel/fax: 0181-251-7912

International Society of Professional Aromatherapists (ISPA)
ISPA House, 82 Ashby Road, Hinckley, Leics LE10 1SN.
tel: 01455-637987; fax: 01455-890956
e-mail: lisabrown@ispa.demon.co.uk

Autogenic Training

British Association for Autogenic Training and Therapy
(BAFATT)
Heath Cottage, Pitch Hill, Ewhurst, nr Cranleigh, Surrey
GU6 7NP.

The British Autogenic Society
Royal London Homoepathic Hospital, Great Ormond Street,
London WC1M 3HR.
tel: 0171-713-6336
website: www.autogenic-therapy.org.uk

Nasim Kanji
Carwood House, 147 Hampermill Lane, Oxhey, Herts
WD1 4PF.
tel: 01923-225402

Bach Flower Remedies

The Dr Edward Bach Centre
Mount Vernon, Sotwell, Oxon OX10 0PZ.
tel: 01491-834678; fax: 01491-825022
e-mail: bach@bachcentre.com; website: www.bachcentre.com
*Services: free help and advice on using the remedies, by tele-
phone, e-mail, fax and letter. Training courses and publi-
cations. Referral to trained, registered practitioners who work
under a strict code of practice.*

Chinese Medicine

The Register of Chinese Herbal Medicine
PO Box 400, Wembley, Middlesex HA9 9NE.
tel: 0181-904-1357
Send an A5 sae (38p stamp) and £2.00 for the register.

Chiropractic

British Chiropractic Association
Blagrave House, 17 Blagrave Street, Reading, Berkshire
RG1 1QB.
tel: 0118-950-5950; fax: 0118-958-8946
e-mail: britchiro@aol.com
website: www.chiropractic-uk.co.uk
*Services: the British Chiropractic Association (BCA) is the
largest association for the chiropractic profession in the UK.
It has been established since 1925, and now represents over
800 UK chiropractors. Amongst the many services it provides
for its members are:*

- *educational programmes and a postgraduate training
  scheme;*
- *a highly effective practice audit service;*
- *strict standards of ethics and conduct;*
- *networks with other professional associations;*
- *medical indemnity insurance.*

*It provides members of the general public with details of their
local chiropractor and can supply packs of leaflets and a
complete register of members for a nominal charge.*

*It takes five years to become a chiropractor at the Anglo-
European College of Chiropractic in Bournemouth, which
offers a BSc degree and postgraduate diploma in chiropractic.
A full time four year BSc course is followed by a postgraduate
year spent on a Vocational Training Scheme (VTS), which
students spend in a chiropractic clinic with the support of a
qualified trainer. Upon successful completion of the VTS the
student is awarded the Diploma in Chiropractic. Glamorgan
University also offers a four year full time BSc (Hons) course,
and Surrey University now runs an MSc course. Only chiropractors trained at an accredited college can become members
of the British Chiropractic Association.*

McTimoney Chiropractic Association
21 High Street, Eynsham, Oxon OX8 1HE.
tel: 01865-880974; fax: 01865-880975
e-mail: admin@mctimoney-chiropractic.org
website: www//mctimoney-chiropractic.org
Services: chiropractic information, directory of practitioners, member services. Send an sae and £5.00 for a register of practitioners.

Colour Therapy

International Association for Colour Therapy
PO Box 3688, London SW13 0NX.
tel: 0181-878-5276

Crystal and Gemstone Therapy

The Affiliation of Crystal Healing Organisations
46 Lower Green Road, Esher, Surrey KT10 8HD.
tel: 0181-398-7252

Cymatics

Dr Sir Peter Manners
Bretforton Hall, Bretforton, Vale of Evesham, Worcestershire WR11 5JH.
tel: 01386-830537; fax: 01386-830918
Services: phone to schedule an appointment at your local cymatics branch in the UK.

Floatation Therapy

The Floatation Association
PO Box 11024, London SW14 7ZF.
Send £1 for a list of UK float centres.

The London Floatation Centre
7A Clapham Common South, London SW4 7AA.
tel: 0171-720-4952

Hellerwork

The European Hellerwork Association
c/o Roger Golten, The MacIntyre Gallery, 29 Crawford Street,
London W1H 1PL.
tel: 0171-723-5676
e-mail: rgolten@dial.pipex.com
website: www.golten.net
For a list of hellerwork practitioners, visit www.heller-work.co.uk
Further information: Golten, R. (1999). The Owners Guide to the Body. London: Thorsons/HarperCollins.

Herbalism

British Herbal Medicine Association
Sun House, Church Street, Stroud GL5 1JL.
tel: 01453-751389
Information leaflets, booklets, compendium, telephone advice.

The General Council and Register of Consultant Herbalists
18 Sussex Square, Brighton, East Sussex BN2 5AA.
tel: 01243-267126

The National Institute of Medical Herbalists
56 Longbrook Street, Exeter EX4 8HA.
tel: 01392-426022

Homoeopathy

British Homoeopathic Association
27A Devonshire Street, London W1N 1RJ.
tel: 0171-935-2163 (1.30–5.30 p.m.)
website: www.nhsconfed.net/bha
Leaflets, referral to medically qualified homoeopathic doctors and veterinary surgeons. Bookshops on premises. Library for the use of members.

Dr Peter Webb
Swan Acre, All Saints Lane, Sutton Courtney, Abingdon, Oxon OX14 4AG.
tel: 01235-848701
Member of the BHA.

The Faculty of Homoeopathy
15 Clerkenwell Close, London EC1R 0AA.
tel: 0171-566 7810; fax: 0171-566-7815

Homoeopathic Trust
15 Clerkenwell Close, London EC1R 0AA.
tel: 0171-566 7800; fax: 0171-566-7815

The Society of Homoeopaths
2 Artizan Road, Northampton NN1 4HU.
tel: 01604-621400; fax: 01604-622622
e-mail: societyofhomoeopaths@btinernet.com
website: www.homoeopathy.org.uk
Send a large sae for a list of practitioners. Has produced an information leaflet, 'Homoeopathy in Pregnancy and Childbirth'.

Hypnotherapy

National Council for Hypnotherapy
Hazelwood, Broadmead, Lymington, Hampshire SO41 6DH.
For a list of qualified therapists in your area, send an sae to:
Bill Broom at the above address.

Leila Hart is qualified in clinical hypnotherapy, deep tissue massage, aromatherapy, yoga stretch and exercise to music. Leila is a lecturer in hypnotherapy and self-hypnosis, and Chairman of the James Braid Society for Clinical Hypnotherapists. She practises in the West End of London. To arrange an appointment, please phone: 0171-402-4311 between 10 a.m. and 7 p.m.

Iridology

Guild of Naturopathic Iridologists
94 Grosvenor Road, London SW1V 3LF.
tel: 0171-821-0255; fax: 0171-821-0255
website: www.gni-International.org
Has a strict code of ethics and comprehensive constitution, protecting the public from the inadequately trained. Provides a register of professionals, who have at least one therapeutic qualification in addition to their iridology diploma, plus professional insurance cover. Provides postgraduate training, biannual newsletter, centre for information. For a register, send an sae.

Janet Spence (iridology, nutritional advice, colon hydrotherapy, manual lymph drainage)

The Complementary Medicine Centre, 20 Coppice Walk, Cheswick Green, Solihull, West Midlands B90 4HY.
tel: 01564-702186

Kinesiology

Association of Systematic Kinesiology
39 Browns Road, Surbiton, Surrey KT5 8ST.
tel: 0181-399-3215; fax: 0181-390-1010
e-mail: info@kinesiology.co.uk
website: www.kinesiology.co.uk
For an extensive list of highly trained registered practitioners, and details of classes, send an A5 envelope and four first class stamps.

For 'Introduction to Kinesiology', a 60 page booklet explaining the basics of AK and featuring the Emotional Stress Release technique please send a cheque for £2.50 (inc. p&p) to TASK Books at the above address. For 'Your Breasts, What Every Woman Needs to Know Now', by Brian Butler, please send a cheque for £10 (inc. p&p) to TASK Books.

Kirlian Photography

The Institute of Kirlian Photographers
51 Rushton Road, Kettering, Northants NN14 2RP.
tel: 01536-762706 (Rosemary Steele); 0181-948-2522 (Felicity Bradley)
Send an sae for a list of acupuncturists who use the technique.

Massage Therapy

Massage Therapy Institute of Great Britain
PO Box 2726, London NW2 4NR.
tel: 0181-208-1607; fax: 0181-208-1639
National register of practitioners and magazine subscription.

London College of Massage
5 Newman Passage, London W1P 3P.
tel: 0171-323-3574; fax: 0171-637-7125

Services: a professional complementary therapy clinic. Mondays to Fridays 9 a.m. to 9 p.m. Pregnancy, labour and baby massage workshops.

Naturopathy

General Council and Register of Naturopaths
Frazer House, 6 Netherall Gardens, London NW3 5RR.
tel: 0171-435-8728

Nutritional Therapy

Dietary Therapy Society
33 Priory Gardens, London N6 5QU.
tel: 0181-341-7260

Society for the Promotion of Nutritional Therapy
PO Box 85, St Albans, Herts. AL3 72Q.
tel: 01582-792088
e-mail: spnt@compuserve.com
website: www.visitweb.com.spnt
Send a large sae plus £1 for a list of your nearest practitioners.

Osteopathy

Osteopathic Information Service
PO Box 2074, Reading, Berkshire RG1 4YR.
tel: 01491-875255

General Council and Register of Osteopaths
56 London Street, Reading, Berkshire RG1 4SQ.
tel: 01734-576585

Reflexology

The British School of Reflexology
Holistic Healing Centre, 92 Sheering Road, Old Harlow, Essex
CM17 0JW.
tel: 01279-429060; fax: 01279-445234
*National practitioner register. Mail order books, charts
and equipment. Training school.* Healing Points—*quarterly
magazine.*

The British Reflexology Association
Monks Orchard, Whitbourne, Worcester WR6 5RB.
tel: 01886-821-207; fax: 01886-822-017
e-mail: bra@britreflex.co.uk; website: www.britreflex.co.uk
*A professional body for reflexology practitioners. Register of
members: £2. Footprints (newsletter): £5 subscription for four
issues. General information leaflet available.*

Reiki

Manjit Ubhi, Reiki Master, 41 Hagley Road, Hayley Green,
Halesowen, West Midlands B63 1DR.
tel: 0121-602-4608

Rolfing

The Rolf Institute Headquarters
206 Canyon Boulevard, Boulder, CO 830 302, USA.

Giselle Genillard, Conversations with Women, 147 Camino
Escondido, Santa Fe, NM 87501, USA.
tel: 001 (505) 989 4662
e-mail: GisGenillard@webtv.net

Spiritual Healing

The National Federation of Spiritual Healers
Old Manor Farm Studio, Church Street, Sunbury-on-Thames,
Middlesex TW16 6RG.
*The NFSH National Healer Referral Service can be reached
Mondays to Fridays 9 a.m.–5 p.m. on 0891-616080 (called
charged at 50p per minute).*

T'ai Chi

The T'ai Chi Union for Great Britain
94 Felsham Road, London SW15 1DQ.
tel: 0181-780-1063
e-mail: cromptonph@aol.com
*Provides contacts, teachers, advice, books, tapes on the sub-
jects of t'ai chi and chi kung (qigong). Mail enquiries must
include a stamped addressed envelope.*

Yoga

British Wheel of Yoga
1 Hamilton Place, Boston Road, Sleaford, Lincolnshire
NG34 7ES.
tel: 01529-306-851; tel/fax: 01529-303233

The Yoga for Health Foundation
Ickwell Bury, Ickwell Green, Bedfordshire SG18 9EF.
tel: 01767-627271; fax: 01767-627266
*Services: a yoga centre, open all year, offering residential
courses for able-bodied and disabled guests. Specially tailored
courses are available for those with MS, ME, asthma, cancer,
arthritis and Parkinson's disease. There are open classes for
local residents, and also training courses for yoga teachers.*

Yoga Biomedical Trust
The Yoga Therapy Centre, Royal London Homoeopathic Hospital, 60 Great Ormond Street, London WC1N 3HR.
tel: 0171-419-7195; fax: 0171-419-7196
e-mail: yogabio.med@virgin.net
website: www.yogatherapy.org
Services: yoga classes—general and specific—for all levels plus pregnancy, postnatal and well-women yoga. Yoga therapy for specific ailments—lower back pain, arthritis, asthma, MS, cancer and elderly people.

US ADDRESSES

Acupuncture

American Association of Acupuncture and Oriental Medicine
4101 Lake Boone Trail Suite 201, Raleigh, NC 27607.
tel: 919-787-5181

National Commission for the Certification of Acupuncturists
PO Box 97075, Washington DC 20090-7075.
tel: 202-232-1404

Traditional Acupuncture Institute
American City Building, Suite 108, Columbia MD 21044.
tel: 410-997-3770

Alexander Technique

North American Society of Teachers of the Alexander Technique
PO Box 517, Urbana, Illinois 61801 0517.
tel: 800 473 0620

Aromatherapy

American Aromatherapy Association
PO Box 3679, South Pasadena, CA 91031.
tel: 818-457-1742

Autogenic Training

Mind Body Health Sciences
393 Dixon Road, Boulder, CO 80302.
tel: 303-440-8460

Bach Flower Remedies

Dr Edward Bach Healing Society
644 Merrick Road, Lynbrook, NY 11563.
tel: 516-593-2206

Chiropractic

American Chiropractic Association
1701 Clarendon Blvd, Arlington, VA 22209.
tel: 703-276-8800

Hellerwork

Hellerwork International
406 Berry Street, Mount Shasta, CA 96067.
tel: 916-926-2500

Herbalism

American Herbalist Guild
PO Box 1683, Soquel, CA 95073.

Homeopathy

National Center for Homeopathy
801 North Fairfax Street, Suite 306, Alexandria, VA 22314.
tel: 703-548-7790

Hypnotherapy

American Institute of Hypnotherapy
1805 E. Garry Ave, Suite 100, Santa Ana, CA 92705.
tel: 714-261-6400

Kinesiology

International College of Applied Kinesiology
PO Box 905, Lawrence, Kansas 66044 0905.
tel: 913-542-1801

Massage

American Massage Therapy Association
820 Davis Street, Suite 100, Evanston, Illinois 60201.
tel: 312-761-2682

Osteopathy

American Osteopathic Association
142 East Ohio Street, Chicago, Illinois 60611.
tel: 312-280-5800

Reflexology

International Institute of Reflexology
PO Box 12642, St Petersburg, Florida 33733.
tel: 813-343-4811

Reiki

Centre for Reiki Training
29209 Northwestern Highway 592, Southfield, Michigan
48034-9841.
tel: 810-948-9534

Rolfing

See US addresses in UK addresses section.

Visualisation

Academy for Guided Imagery
PO Box 2070, Mill Valley, CA 94942.
tel: 415-389-9324

Yoga

International Association of Yoga Therapists
109 Hillside Ave, Mill Valley, CA 94941.
tel: 415-383-4587

General

Allied and Alternative Medicine online database (AMED)
http://www.rs/ch/wwv/rs/ds/amed.html

Alternative Medicine Homepage (University of Pittsburgh)
http://www.pitt.edu/~cbw/altm.html

American College of Obstetricians and Gyneologists Resource
Center
409 12th Street NW, Washington, DC 20024-2188.
tel: 202-638-5577

American Holistic Medical Association
4101 Lake Boone Trail, Suite 201, Raleigh, NC 27607.
tel: 919-787-5181

National Association of Child-Bearing Centers
3123 Gottschall Road, 1518 Perkiomenville, PA 18074.
tel: 215-234-8068

National Clearinghouse for Alcohol and Drug Information
PO Box 2345, Rockville, MD 20847-2345.
tel: 301-468-2600 or 800-729-6686

National Women's Health Network
514 10th Street NW, Washington DC 20004.
tel: 202-347-1140

National Women's Health Resource Center
Suite 325, 2440 M St NW, Washington DC 20037.
tel: 202-293-6045

Office of Alternative Medicine Information Center
National Institutes of Health, Suite 450, 6120 Executive Blvd,
Rockville, MD 20892-9904.
tel: 301-402-2466

Office on Smoking and Health
Mail Stop K-50, Atlanta, GA 30333.
Smoking, tobacco and health information line: 800-232-1311

Society for Nutrition Education
2001 Kilebrew Drive, Suite 340, Minneapolis MN 55425.
tel: 612-854-0035

Index